Dress Like a Million Bucks...

While Spending Only Pennies!

An Insider's Guide
to finding Designer Bargains at
Drop-Dead Prices in New York

**Includes
Listings for:**
New York City
Long Island
Westchester
W. Connecticut

PAMELA PARISI
The Elegant Tightwad

© 2002 by Pamela Parisi

ISBN 1-59196-033-9

This book is dedicated to my Aunt Mae, from whom I inherited the bargain-hunting gene and to my Mom and Dad, for teaching me the value of a dollar.

Part2/ Pre-owned Clothing/57

Introduction

I saw the ad in New York Magazine. But, oh no! I would have only 1 hour to shop between getting home from school and going to work. I ran to the sale and, as usual, there was a long line. By the time I made it to the front it was time to leave. I was crushed. However they assured me that the stock was so extensive I would certainly find something great tomorrow. I left disappointed but hopeful that what they told me was true.

When I awoke the next morning everything was still and white. And covered with 18 inches of snow! While the city slept it was hit with the biggest blizzard New York had seen in many years. Did that deter me in my quest? Please! Don't insult me. I layered up and set out to brave the elements. No taxis or buses running? No problem. I'll just walk. I inched through the snow, bundled up like Nanook of the north, wind slicing at my face, with visions of below wholesale price tags dancing in my head. After my long and arduous trek (well, 3 blocks actually), I arrived at my destination. A lone maintenance man was the only human to be seen for miles, or at least a block. He looked at me with amazement and asked, *"What* are you doing here?" I answered, "Well, there's this really great sale today." The look of shock and incredulity on his face gave way to knowing amusement. As he smiled and shook his head, he uttered, "You gals'll do anyting fer a sale."

Yes! We will! Well, on second thought maybe not *anything.* But we'll go pretty damn far.

Was it worth it? You bet! I found some of the most memorable bargains of my life at this sale. And what it took to get them made it so much sweeter. Sure, finding great deals on the sale racks at Bloomingdales is nice. But to me, that's like going on a safari in a zoo. *That's* for sissies! The *thrill of the hunt* is my motivation. There is no greater pleasure than bagging an Armani suit or a pair of Ferragamo shoes at 50% below wholesale. Oh, all right. If the truth were told, I guess there is at least *one* greater pleasure. Can you imagine experiencing both of those in one twenty-four hour period? Hallelujah brother! That is a *blessed* day. But that's a subject for another book.

This book is about shopping, specifically, bargain shopping. It's a directory of where to find great designer clothes at drop-dead prices. The sale that I'd mentioned previously happened over 20 years ago. In the ensuing period of time I have become an expert at routing out the best sales and stores and events at which you can find great clothes for a fraction of their intended retail prices. I have listings in this book for everything from sample sales, to off-price stores and showrooms, to consignment and thrift shops. Whether your taste runs to Versace and Fendi, or Banana Republic and Gap; whether you want only the trendiest current season styles or are looking for a classic Chanel from the 40's, you can find the places to get them in this book.

When I decided to compile these resources I knew my knowledge was extensive. In researching this book, I found so much more than I could ever have imagined. We have the good luck to be located in New York, the fashion capital of the world. There is more opportunity to find the best clothing at the lowest prices here, than anywhere else.

Almost all of the top designers have showrooms in New York. What this means for us is that sample sales will occur right here. What's a sample sale, you ask? Every season a designer creates a new line of clothing. Samples are made of that line for salesmen to show to buyers all over the country and the world. Fall samples are shown during the previous spring, and spring samples during the previous fall. So when the actual season is upon us, these samples, which are not *technically* new, can be sold. Hence a sample sale. Prices are usually at wholesale and below, sometimes sinfully below, and it is the merchandise

2

that is currently available in stores. A true sample sale will have only one size, usually 6-8, however many sample sales also have overstock, so other sizes are available.

Which brings us to another benefit to having the designers right in our backyard. Overstock. When orders are taken for the new line, there is a certain amount of the clothing manufactured over that required to fill the orders. This is overstock. You'll find this merchandise everywhere from off-price retail stores to consignment and thrift shops, to special charity events. The prices will make you swoon!

There are those who will only buy brand, spanking new duds and others, like myself, who will follow the whiff of a great bargain anywhere it may lead. I love trolling for treasures at consignment and thrift stores. Having been to them at every place I have *ever* visited or lived, I can say without equivocation that New York has the best. You'll find the most current and gently used items imaginable and at prices that might inspire you to drop to your knees and praise Allah. In addition to used items, you can find many new things in these shops, either donated, as is the case in not-for-profit thrift shops or sold to, as is the case in consignment shops.

I have visited quite a large number of the stores listed in this directory. At the time of printing all of the information, such as address, store hours, etc., was accurate. Remember that the examples of stock and prices are what *were* available at *that* time. Although this will give you an idea of the types of items carried and their prices, it does not guarantee that that particular item will be there when you shop. All discount establishments, from thrift shops to department stores, get what is available to them at any given time. They're not akin to regular retail stores, which orders their stock months and months in advance. And herein lies the exquisite joy of bargain shopping – it's a treasure hunt. When you head out loaded for bear, you never know what you'll find.

And before I close, let me say a few words about myself. Clothes are a passion. I began designing clothing at age 13 and did have my own small manufacturing company for 8 years. I wore many hats as the owner of this company. None brought me more joy than that of designer. During my more youthful years, I worked in New York's garment district as a showroom model, so I have participated in the fashion industry from many angles.

My bargain hunting "career" also began during my teen years, having been taken to my first "bag sale" at the age of 16. Coming home with a bag full of clothes for which I paid $1 was all I needed. I was hooked! I have never broken the habit, just simply perfected it. This book combines my passion for clothes with my passion for bargain hunting and the result is a product that I have had enormous fun both researching and writing. I hope you will have as much fun using this guide. But enough chit-chat...

Let's go shopping!

Pamela Parisi – The Elegant Tightwad
April 29, 2002

Part 1

New Clothing
ϛϛϛϛϛϛϛϛ

Sample Sales
Showrooms
Sale Events
Retail Stores(Individual)
Retail Chain Stores
Outlet Centers

___Chapter 1 ___

Sample Sales & Showrooms

Every season a designer creates a new line of clothing. Samples are made of that line for salesmen to show buyers all over the country and the world. Fall samples are shown during the previous spring, and spring samples during the previous fall. So when the actual season is upon us, these samples, which are not *technically* new, can be sold. Hence a sample sale. Prices are usually wholesale and below, and it is the current merchandise that you are seeing in the stores. They are held either right in the showroom or at a location rented out for the purpose of this event. A true sample sale will have only one size, usually 6-8, however many sample sales also have overstock, so other sizes are available. Be sure to call and check if your size will be available, if that information is not posted

You can stroll down 7th Avenue, between 34th and 42nd streets on any weekday and be handed flyers announcing sample sales that are going on. There are lots of other ways to find out about them though. I have listed showroom/warehouse spaces that host sample sales on a permanent or semi-permanent basis. These will have mailing lists you can be added onto for alerts of upcoming events. There are listings in magazines, subscription newsletters and on websites, the latter of which will also compile mailing lists that you can be added to. Some are held at hotels or exhibition spaces. Whenever you go to one of these sales, always ask if they have a mailing list and sign up.

Shopping at sample sales is a bit different from sashaying through Macy's on a Saturday afternoon. Most of the time there is a line waiting to get in. Get there early for the best selection. Wear comfortable clothes with a body suit or the like underneath. No where is the admonition from our mothers to wear good undies more applicable. Most don't have dressing rooms, so if you are allowed to try garments on leave your inhibitions behind.

I always wear a fanny pack, so that I have both hands free. You want to be able to rip through the clothing at lightning speed. Don't dawdle, if you snooze you loose. That great cashmere sweater will be snatched up, if not right out of your hands, if you pause to breathe. Yes Virginia, there are "aggressive shoppers" out there. Don't be intimidated by them! Hold your ground and think of it as football for females. Which brings us to the other reason for having both hands free. You will want to be able to slap back any item pulled out of your hands, if on principle only. Am I exaggerating? Oh, of course I am! But just a little.

Manhattan

Project
175 Orchard St. (Statton & Houston)
212-505-0500

M-Sun. 11-7

This store/showroom holds sample sales on an ongoing basis. The stock changes every two weeks and most lines will be there once per year. Some of the designers that sell their samples at this location are Armani, Valentino, Stephane Kelian, and Franco Ferre. The sizes range from 2-12, however most of the merchandise is sizes 6-8. To be put on their mailing list and receive email alerts send a message to assaf@inch.com

A Nice Price/SSS Sample Sale
261 W. 36th St., 2nd Floor
212-947-8748 (Hotline)

This is a showroom /warehouse that runs sample and stock sales on an ongoing basis. You can call their hotline or access them online at http://www.clothingline.com for information on the current sales. Prices are at wholesale and below. You can be added to their mailing list simply by clicking "Mailing List" on their website and you will receive schedules of weekly sales.

They also have a retail store, Nice Price, at 493 Columbus Ave, between 83rd & 84th streets.

Collective Elite
560 7th Ave.

This showroom has between 30 and 40 sales per year. To get the skinny on these events write to Collective Elite, P.O. Box 1631, New York, NY 10150 or email debra@aol.com and you will be added to their mailing list.

Media

In New York Magazine check out the "Sales and Bargains" column and in Time Out New York it's the "Shop Talk" column. They list the current week's sample sales in addition to other sale events. New York Magazine also has this info available online. See listing below for web address.

Websites for Sample Sales

Bargain Hotline
http://www.bargainhotline.com - This is a site you can subscribe to for weekly updates of showroom, sample and warehouse sales. A yearly subscription is $40 and this includes current

listings of sales, sent every Friday, and last minute updates throughout the week, all delivered directly to your email address

New York Sale
http://www.nysale.com – This is a free subscription site you can access for sample, showroom, warehouse and retail store sales and events. You will receive weekly updates of current sales in your email box along with intermittent sale alerts.

New York Magazine
http://nymetro.com/shopping/articles/sb/index.htm - This will take you to the magazine's "Sales and Bargains" column. Sales are updated here on a daily basis and you can sign up for email alerts. On the left hand panel click "Newsletter Signup" and then click "Best Bets" to be added to their mailing list.

Daily Candy
http://www.dailycandy.com – This website has listings of sales and other events. You can subscribe and get alerts emailed to you.

Individual Designers

Chaiken
212-334-3501

You'll find an assortment of goods from this women's better sportswear line. They're famous for their great fitting pants and you can grab them at below wholesale prices at these sales. You'll find pants which retail for $200 for $80 and sweaters which go for $115 in the stores for $45-$50. They happen twice yearly, in May and November, at changing locations. The original samples are size 4 and the stock is sizes 0-12. You can call the showroom for the sale dates and location.
Visa, MC and Amex are accepted.

Dosa
212-431-1733

Their twice-yearly sample sales are held in February and August This line is designed by Christina Kim and features the lingerie look and layering. You'll find skirts with matching pants, to be worn together, Chinese jackets and those interesting rumpled silk skirts. Garments which retail for $95-$500 can be grabbed here for $20-$250. The location of the sales change, so call to be put on their mailing list.

Onward Kashiyama
1 E. 27th St.
212-629-6100

This showroom has sales in November and May. Some of the designers you will find are Michael Kors, Paul Smith, Alexander McQueen, Peplem and Chuck Roaste. You'll pay wholesale prices for this great stuff and you can call and be put on their mailing list to get your invitation.

TSE
917-606-6700

At these sales, which are held in April or May and October or November you'll find TSE, TSE Say and TSE Men. Prices are 30% below wholesale and lower. The locations of the sales change, so you can call a month before to find out all the pertinent information.

Vera Wang
@ Hotel Pennsylvania
401 Seventh Ave., 18th Fl.
212-575-6400

If you're looking to walk down the aisle in style, this is the place for you. These sample sales are held twice a year, in April and October, at the Hotel Pennsylvania. It can be an accomplishment just finding out the dates of these events. My suggestion would be to call the hotel directly, as the showroom is not terribly delighted to receive these inquiries. Make sure you arrive well before the posted time, because the competition for these great wedding gowns, bridesmaid dresses, and evening gowns can be fierce. Prices are at wholesale and below.

Meg Cohen
920 Broadway (20th&21st)
Suite 905
212-473-4002

These sales are held 3 times a year, in December, February and May. You'll find Meg's beautiful English cashmere scarves, throws, and blankets. Prices are at wholesale and below. Scarves which sell for $175 in stores you can grab here for between $50-$80. Call the showroom for dates and times.

Miriam Haskell
49 W. 37th St. (5th&6th)
 212-764-3332

This sale is held once a year in December. Although you may have to search for Haskell's designs from the 40's and 50's at vintage shops and flea markets, you can get the company's current pieces here for a song. Prices start at $10 and they are always at wholesale and below. Call the showroom to be added to their mailing list.

Portolano
32 W. 39th St. (5th&6th)
5th Fl.
212-719-4403

You find gloves by Portolano for Fendi and Moschino, cashmere sweaters, handbags, small leather items and pashmina shawls at these sales. They're held in October, November and December and you can call the showroom for the dates. Prices are at wholesale, which for these items is 60% off the retail price.

Norma Kamali
11 W. 56th St. (5th&6th)
212-852-6254

You'll have to call for the dates of these sales, but if you love Norma Kamali, you won't be disappointed. Expect lots of surprises and fabulous prices.

Nanette Lapore
225 W. 35th St. (7th&8th)
212-594-0012

These sales happens 4 times a year in her design
studio. They go on for 3 days and it is rumored
that there is even a dressing room. Yikes! Prices
are at wholesale and way below. Call for
information.

___Chapter 2____

Sale Events

Barney's Warehouse Sale
(212) 929-9000

We love this store anytime! But during this fabulous sale, which is held twice a year, we are delirious about it. You'll find the great merchandise that you see at Barney's throughout the season priced at whopping discounts. Call for dates and location

Prasad's Beyond Fashion Sale
Milk Studios
450 West 15th Street, 2nd Floor
(9th and 10th Avenue)
NYC
http://www.beyondfashion.org

This is an event to die for! This incredible sale and auction is held once a year in NYC, during late May/early June. It begins with a preview night featuring both a silent and live auction, and *of course*, shopping the racks. Some of the great items auctioned off this year were: The Beyond Fabulous Makeover Package - by Stylists to the

Stars, a $21,000 Amanpuri Beach Resort Vacation in Phuket, Thailand, a Maggie Norris Evening Dress and Gown and Dinner for Six with House & Garden's Lora Zarubin and Jay McInerney.

The clothing sale starts right after the auction and continues on for the next four days. It includes shoes and accessories in addition to the clothes, donated by literally hundreds of designers, all priced well below wholesale. What is wonderful about this sale is that new merchandise arrives daily, so you can go every day and find new surprises. The list of designers is far too extensive to include here, however I will give you some examples of what I saw. A Donna Karen tan soft wool sweater $60, Dolce and Gabanna pants $230, Calvin Klein skirts and dresses $40-$55, Versace pants $148-$228, an Yves St. Laurent white cotton jacket sporting a $1500 price tag just $400 here. There were lots of jeans; Comme de Garcon $45, Cambrio $48, Bill Blass $40 and Marc Jacobs $150. Tocca dresses, skirts and tops were $15-$125 and Hanky Panky cute stretch tops were $15. This just scratches the surface.

All of this and you can also shop without guilt! Hell, go ahead and splurge, because all proceeds go to a wonderful cause. By shopping at PRASAD's Beyond Fashion sale, you can help to change the lives of needy children and their families around the world. The Prassad Project (Philantropic Relief/Altruistic Service and

Development) is a humanitarian organization started during the 1930's to provide relief for children and families living in poverty throughout rural India. It has expanded greatly over the years and now provides aid to the underprivileged in Mexico and the USA.

The preview night is $75 admission and sale days are &15. The location up to now has been the Milk Studios, but that could change in the future, so make sure to check on that. For info you can call 845-434-0376 about one month before, or visit their website http://www.prasad.org

Shoe-Inn Semi-Annual Warehouse Sale
@Parsons School of Design Exhibition Space
66 5th Ave.
NYC
&
@American Legion Hall
Route 27 (across from Brents)
Amagansett
877-746-3466

Imelda Marcos would have to be revived if she walked through the door of this event! There are over 12,000 pairs of current season shoes and boots to choose from, all of them marked down 30-50% from their original retail prices. They also carry handbags, belts, wallets, hair accessories and more. You'll find Kate Spade, Michael Kors,

Stuart Weitzman, Ann Klein, Donald Pliner and Tayran Rose, to name just a few of the hundreds of designers available. Joan Hamburg has called this the "event of the season." It's held every January in NYC and every August in Amagansett. It runs for 10 days and you can call to be added to their mailing list.

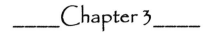

_____Chapter 3_____

Retail Stores (Individual)

These stores carry designer clothing, shoes, accessories, etc., at discount prices. Not to be confused with discount stores like Kohl's or the like, this is current designerwear sold off-price. The stock varies, as do the markdowns and, as in most stores, certain types of styles will prevail. Get added to the mailing lists where available and always ask if they have any type of special promotions or regular shoppers discount cards.

Long Island

Huntington

Designer Outlet
1200-1 E. Jericho Tpk.
631-271-5711

T-Sat. 10:30-6

This small store may be the only one of it's kind on Long Island, in that it is an individual off price shop. Their stock consists of samples and overstock from many of the upscale stores and designers we love   All items are current season and at 50%-80% off the retail price You may find Ralph Lauren, Ann Klein, Ungaro, Donna Karan and Iceberg. Bloomingdales and Saks will unload overstock here, so many of the labels that you will see at those establishments sometimes make their way to these racks. They also get wedding dresses, great handbags and jewelry from time to time. Some of the incredible deals that I have seen include Ralph Lauren tops which retail for $98 for $25, a $490 Ann Klein suit for $165, Liz jeans for $25 and a $3500 wedding gown priced at $500. The Inca straw bags that you see at Nordstrom for $90 are a mere $10 here. Stock changes rapidly, so what you find today may not be there tomorrow, however fantastic bargains are always available. Major credit cards and checks are accepted.

Manhattan

Designer's Promise
93 Nassau St.
 (212) 227-4454

M-F 9:30-7:30

You find women's designer clothing here priced at least 50% below the normal retail value. Some of the names they carry are Ann Klein, Donna Karan and Westcott.

Fishkin Knitwear
314 Grand St. (Allen)
(212) 226-6538

M-Th. 10-5
F 10-4
Sun. 9-4:30

This store carries women's better sportswear, bathing suits and shoes. They specialize in cashmere for women and prices can range from 20%-70% less than normal retail. Some of the names you will see are Eileen Fisher, Adrienne Vittadini and Sarah Arizona.

All major credit cards and checks are accepted.

Designer Warehouse
600 Broadway   (Houston & Broadway)
2nd Fl.

12 East 14th St. (5th & Broadway)
(212) 239-7272

515 Broadway (Spring & Broome)
(212) 334-1152

M-Sun. 11-7

These stores carry luxury brand names such as
Fendi, Prada, Dolce & Gabanna and Deisel. Some
recent finds were D & G dresses retailing at $399
on sale for $99. Diesel pants retailing at $115 -
$140 on sale for $39, Fendi FF jackets retailing at
$1400 on sale $299 - $399; Fendi pants retailing
at $350 on sale $99 and Diesel T-shirts retailing at
$45 on sale for $12. Sizes available from 0 – 12

Visa, MC and Amex accepted.

Find Outlet
361 W. 17th St. (8th & 9th)
212-243-3177
Th.-Sun. 12-7

229 Mott St. (Prince & Spring)
212-226-5167
M-Sun. 12-7

This is an off-price outlet for trendoids. You'll
find the some of same clothes you see at Barney's,
Scoop and Intermix here for 50%-80% off their
regular retail prices. Some of the names you'll
come across are Marc by Marc Jacobs, Anna Sui,
Tufi Duek, Mint, Dolce & Gabanna, Katayone
Adeli and Jill Stuart.   They carry sizes 0-12. Their
stock changes on a daily basis, so email them at
findout@findoutlet.com and get on their mailing
list for updates.

Visa, MC accepted.

Canal Jeans
504 Bdwy (Broome & Spring)
212-226-1130

M-Sun. 9:30-9

This discount department store, with 5 full floors,
is the largest store in Soho. You'll find men's and
women's clothing and shoes, and lingerie ranging
from the traditional to the trendy to the funky.
They carry Calvin Klein, Polo and Levi's among
others and the have the largest selection of jeans in

New York. There is also a vintage department with items from the 1940's to 1970's.

Major credit cards, personal and traveler's checks are accepted.

Gabay's
225 1st Ave. (13th & 14th)
212-254-3180

M-Sun. 10-8

This is a small store just chock full of great deals. The designer clothes that you will find at this store are both regular and seconds, at 70% off the normal retail price. Some of the designers they carry on a consistent basis are Armani, DKNY, Gucci, Fendi, Ralph Lauren and Dolce & Gabanna. Prices can range anywhere from $25-$600

Major credit cards are accepted.

A Nice Price
493 Columbus Ave. (83rd & 84th)
212-362-1020

M-Sat. 11-7
Sun. 12-6

This is an off-price clothing store carrying contemporary styles. They carry sizes 2-12 at 60%-70% off the regular retail price. Some of the names you'll see here are Theory, Essendi, White & Warren and Fay Joseph.

Brooklyn

Aaron's
627 5th Ave. (17th)
718-768-5400

M-Sat. 9:30-6
Th. till 9

This 10,000 square foot store carries women's upscale clothing and accessories at 30% off the regular retail price. You'll find most designers, including Max Mara, Ann Ferre, Dana Buchman, Hugo Boss, Eileen Fisher, Ann Klein, Jones NY and Isda & Co. They carry all sizes from 2-20. Although this is an off-price establishment, the type of service you'll receive there makes it feel more like an upscale boutique. There are no minimums for the dressing room and they have a waiting area for husbands and kids complete with couches, TVs and DVDs. They provide coffee, tea, espresso and cookies free of charge and there is also a free parking lot for customers right across the street.
MC, Visa, Amex, and Discover are accepted.

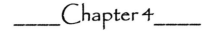

_____Chapter 4_____

Retail Stores (Chains)

Some of these chains have very familiar names, with stores throughout the country. Others like Forman's, Fox's or Century 21 are more of a New York phenomenon and may not be as well known. The latter I have listed to give you a heads up on these great places, the former mainly to provide the locations of the stores throughout this area

Long Island

Century 21
1085 Old Country Road   (Exit W2 Wantagh
Parkway)
Wesbury
(516) 333-5200

M-Sat: 10 -9:30
Sun: 11-7

This store, which calls itself "NYC's best kept
secret", now has a Long Island location. In
addition to off-price designer fashions, you can
find shoes, lingerie, linens, cosmetics, accessories
handbags, luggage, housewares, giftware and
electronics. Prices are always 40%-70% off
regular retail and you can find many of the fashion
forward designs that you see in top New York
stores.

Daffy's
They offer a wide selection of apparel and
accessories for men, women, and children. You'll
find designer collections and brand names at up to
80% off the regular retail price. Their website is at
http://www.daffys.com.

Manhasset
Northern Boulevard   (Next to Americana Mall)
516 -365-4477
M-F 10 - 9
Sat. 10 – 6
Sun. 12 - 6

Smithtown
20 E. Main Street
516 265-4477
M-W 10 - 7
Th-F 10 – 9
Sat. 10 – 7
Sun. 12 – 6

Fox's
You'll find designer clothing here for gals ranging
from teens to mature ladies and casual to
eveningwear.   Prices are less than 50% of regular
retail. Most of the labels are cut out of the clothes,
however some are left in. This is all current
season merchandise and they carry sizes 2-14.

Mineola
80 Main Street
516- 294-8321

Huntington
12 Elm Street
516- 424-5221

M, T, W & Sat. 10-6
Th. & F 10-8
Sun. 12-5

Loehmann's
This store has been selling upscale women's
clothing off price since 1921 Their Back Room is
where the action is, with top designer names
selling for 30-65% off of the regular retail price.
They now also carry shoes and accessories,
juniors, fragrances, gifts and intimate apparel.
Some of their stores even have a men's
department. Be sure to join the "Insider's Club"
for special discounts and sale alerts. You can visit
them online at http://www.loehmanns.com.

Hewlett
1296 Broadway
516-374-5195

Huntington
301 W. Jericho Tpk.
631-423-2020

M-F 10-9
Sat. 10-7
Sun. 11-6

New Hyde Park
1550 Union Tpk.
516-328-8900

M-Sat. 10-9
Sun. 11-6

Sym's
60 Vanderbilt Motor Pkwy
Commack NY
631-864-9600
M-F 10 – 9
Sat. 10 - 6
Sun. 12 – 5

695 Merrick Pkwy
Westbury
516-683-0018
M-F 10 – 9
Sat. 10 – 6
Sun. 11 – 5

TJ Maxx
This is the largest off-price retail clothing chain in
the United States. You'll find brand name family
apparel, giftware, domestics, women's shoes,
accessories and fine jewelry at 20-60% below
department store prices. Check out their website at
http://www.tjmaxx.com.

M-Sat. 9:30-9:30
Sun. 11-6

Massapequa
5500 Sunrise Highway
516-799-5201

Hicksville
410 South Oyster Bay Road
516-433-4880

Carle Place
217 Glen Cove Rd
516-462-2610

Commack
5020 Jericho Turnpike
631-462-2610

Oceanside
3221 Long Beach Road
516-766-8110

Manhattan

Forman's

You'll find women's better clothing and accessories at these stores. They sell their merchandise at 20%-60% less than the regular retail price. You'll find Jones NY, Liz Claiborne, Gianni and Rena Rowan among others, on a regular basis. In addition to regular sized items, they also have petite and plus size departments.

Visa, MC, Amex, Discover and checks are accepted.

82 Orchard St. (Grand & Broome)
212-228-2500
Sun.-W 9-6
Th. 9-8
F 9-4

59 John St. (William)
212-791-4100
M-W 8-7
Th. 8-8
F 8-4

145 E. 42nd St. (Lex. & 3rd)
212-681-9800

560 5th Ave. (46th)
212-719-1000
M-Th. 8-8
F 8-4
Sun. 10-6

Bolton's
You'll find lower end designer and brand name
career fashions and sportswear, accessories and
lingerie at these shops.

90 Broad St.
212-785-0513
M-W 8-6
Th. & F 8:30-7

1180 Madison Ave.
212-722-4419
M-F 10-8
Sat. 10-7
Sun. 12-6

4 East 34th St.
212-684-3750
M, T & F 10-8
W & Th. 9-8
Sat. 10-7
Sun. 11-6

111 West 51st St.
212-245-5227
M-F 8-6:30
Sat. & Sun. 10-6

Century 21
22 Cortlandt Street
212-227-9092

M-W & F 7:45am to 8pm
Th: 7:45-8:30
Sat: 10-8
Sun 11-7

Daffy's
335 Madison Ave. (44th St.)
212-557-4422
M-F 8-8
Sat. 10-6
Sun. 12-6

125 E. 57th St. (Park Ave.)
212-376-4477
M-F 10-8
Sat. 10-7
Sun. 12-6

1311 Broadway (34th St.)
212-736-4477
M-F 10-9
Sat. 10-8

Sun. 11-7

111 Fifth Ave. (18th St.)
212-529-4477
M-Sat. 10-9
Sun. 12-6

462 Broadway (Grand St.)
212-334-7444
M-Th. 10:30-8
F-Sun. 10:30-9

Loehmann's
101 7th Ave. (16th St.)
212-352-0856

M-Sat. 9-9
Sun. 11-7

Sym's
400 Park Ave.
212-317-8200

M- F 10 - 7:30
Sat. 10 - 6
Sun. 12 - 5

42 Trinity Pl.
(212)797-1199
M- W 9 - 6

Th. - F 9 - 8
Sat. 10 - 6
Sun. 12 - 5

TJ Maxx
620 Ave. Of The Americas (18th & 19th)
212-229-0875
M-Sat 9:30-9
Sun. 11-7

Brooklyn

Fox's
923 Kings Highway
Brooklyn, NY 11223
(718) 645-3620

M-Sat. 10-6
Th. till 8
Sun. 11-6

Century 21
472 86th St. (4th & 5th)
(718) 748-3266

M-W & F 10-8
Th. 10-9
Sat. 10-9:30
Sun. 11-7

Loehmann's
Sheepshead Bay
Loehmann's Seaport Plaza
2807 E. 21st St.
(718) 368-1256

M-Sat. 10-10
Sun. 11-6

Queens

Daffy's
Queens Blvd (55th & 56th)
718 760-7787
M-Sat. 10-9:30
Sun. 11-7

TJ Maxx
College Point
136-05 20th Avenue
718-353-2727

M-Sat. 9:30-9:30
Sun. 11-7

Staten Island

TJ Maxx
1509 Forest Avenue
718-876-1995

2530 Hylan Boulevard
718-980-4150

M-Sat. 9:30-9:30
Sun. 11-6

Bronx & Westchester

Fox's
Eastchester
15 Waverly Place
914-793-1573
M-Sat. 10-6
Th. till 8
Sun. 12-5

Sym's
Elmsford
395 Tarrytown Rd.
914-592-2447

Riverdale
5740 Broadway
718-543-6420

White Plains
29 Tarrytown Rd.
914-948-8090

M-F 10-9
Sat. 10-8:30
Sun. 12-5:30

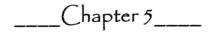

_____Chapter 5_____

Outlet Centers

I have included primarily clothing stores in this list. There are other types of merchandise available at these centers. Please visit the websites or call the mall directly for this information.

Long Island

The Mall at the Source
Westbury
1504 Old Country Rd. (Elison Rd.)
(516) 228-0303

M-Sat. 10-9:30
Sun. 11-6

This mall has regular and outlet stores. Listed here are the outlets. You can call the mall to be connected directly to any store.

Ann Taylor Loft
Nordstrom Rack
Off 5th-Saks Fifth Avenue Outlet
L'eggs Hanes Bali Playtex Factory Outlet

Pacific Sunwear Outlet
Rosewood Home Furnishing Outlet
The Children's Place Outlet
Wilsons Leather Outlet

Prime Outlets at Bellport
Bellport
10 Farber Drive
http://primeoutlets.com/p.cfm/centers/Bellport
631-286-4952

January & February
M-Th. 10-6
F & Sat. 10-9
Sun. 11-6

March – December
M-Sat. 10-9
Sun. 11-6

Bass Outlet
Dress Barn/Dress Barn Woman
Gap Outlet
Geoffrey Beene
L'eggs, Hanes, Bali, Playtex
Liz Claiborne
Lorianna
Maidenform
Pendleton
Rue 21 Company Store

VF Factory Outlet
Van Heusen Direct
Bugle Boy
Nautica
The Jockey Store
Little Big Dogs
Nike Factory Store
Reebok Factory Store
T-Shirts Plus
Banister Shoe Studio
Dexter Shoe
Easy Spirit
Famous Footwear
Marty's Shoes
Natuaralizer Outlet
Nine West
Van's Shoes

Tanger Outlet Center
Riverhead
Tanger Drive, Suite 200 (I-495 East, Long Island
Expressway Exit 72)
http://www.tangeroutlet.com/
800-407-4894
631-369-2732
M-Sat. 9-9
Sun. 10-8

Aeropostale
Ann Taylor Loft
Banana Republic Factory Store

Barney's New York
Bass Clothing & Shoe Outlet
BCBG
Benetton
Big Dog Sportswear
Brooks Brothers
California Sunshine Swimwear
Calvin Klein
Casual Corner
Casual Corner Woman
Casual Male Big & Tall Outlet
Claiborne Men's
Club Monaco
Cutter & Buck
Dana Buchman
Danskin
Delia's
DKNY Jeans
Donna Karan
Dress Barn
Dress Barn Woman
Eddie Bauer
Elisabeth
Gap Outlet
Geoffrey Beene
Greg Norman Golf Outlet
Guess?
Haggar Clothing Co.
Izod
J. Crew
Jockey

Jones New York
Jones New York Sport
Joseph Abboud
Kasper
L'eggs Hanes Bali Playtex
L'eggs Hanes Bali Playtex Express
Levi's Outlet by Designs
Liz Claiborne Outlet
London Fog
Maidenform
Maternity Works
Nautica
Nike
OFF 5TH Saks Fifth Avenue Outlet
Old Navy Outlet
Olga Warner
Pacific Sunwear
Perry Ellis
Petite Sophisticate
Polo Jeans Co. Factory Store
Polo Ralph Lauren Factory Store
Rave Girl
Reebok Outlet Store
Rena Rowan
Rue 21
Socks Galore by Hanes
Tommy Hilfiger
Van Heusen
Woolrich

Upstate

Woodbury Common Premium Outlets
Central Valley
498 Red Apple Court
845-928-4000
http://premiumoutlets.com/

Mon-Sat 10-9, Sun 10-8

This outlet center stands out in that it has all of the
very top names in fashion represented. You'll find
Chanel, Chrisian Dior, Fendi, Prada, Eileen Fisher,
Dolce & Gabanna, just to name a few. It's only an
hour from the city and very easy to get to. You
can call the main phone number to be connected to
any store.

A|X Armani Exchange
Adidas
Andrew Marc
Ann Taylor Factory Store
Anne Klein
Arden B.
Avenue
Banana Republic Factory Store
Barneys New York Outlet
Bass
BCBG Max Azria
Bebe
Benetton

Betsey Johnson
Big Dog Sportswear
Bottega Veneta
Brooks Brothers Factory Store
Burberry
Calvin Klein
Carolina Herrera   Spring 2002
Casual Corner
Chanel
Christian Dior
Cinzia Rocca
Claiborne Menswear
Club Monaco
Dana Buchman
Danskin
Delia's
DKNY Jeans
DNA Easyway
Dolce & Gabbana
Donna Karan
Dress Barn
Eddie Bauer
Eileen Fisher
Elisabeth
Ellen Tracy
Escada Company Store
Etro
Fendi
Fila
French Connection
FUBU

Gap Outlet
Geoffrey Beene
Giorgio Armani General Store
Greg Norman
Gucci
Guess
Harve Benard
Hugo Boss
Iceberg Factory Store
Izod
J. Crew
Jockey
Jones New York
Jones New York Country
Jones New York Mens & Womens Suits
Jones New York Sport
Jones New York Woman
Joseph Abboud
Kasper ASL
Kenneth Cole
L'eggs Hanes Bali Playtex
La Perla
Lacoste
Levi's Outlet by Designs
Liz Claiborne
London Fog
Louis Feraud
Lucky Brand Jeans   Summer 2002
Maidenform
Malo
Marina Rinaldi

Max Mara
Natori
Nautica
Nautica Jeans
Neiman Marcus Last Call
Nike Factory Store
The North Face
Off 5th - Saks Fifth Avenue Outlet
Oilily
PacSun
A Pea in the Pod
Perry Ellis
Petite Sophisticate
Polo Jeans Co. Factory Store
Polo Ralph Lauren Factory Store
Puma   Summer 2002
Quiksilver
Reebok
Salvatore Ferragamo
Space (Prada, Miu Miu)
St. John Company Store
Studio 7 (Celine, Loewe, Christian Lacroix)
Studio 7 (Marc Jacobs, Givenchy, Michael Kors)
Tahari
Theory
Timberland
Tommy Hilfiger
TSE
Van Heusen
Variazioni
Versace

Wilsons Leather Outlet
Wolford
Woolrich
XOXO
Zegna Outlet Store

—Part 2—
Pre-Owned Clothing
ϚϚϚϚϚϚ

Consignment Shops
Thrift Shops
Special Sale Events
Vintage Shops
Vintage Sale Events
Chain Thrift Shops

_____Chapter 6_____

Consignment & Thrift Shops

Consignment shops carry primarily used items, however you will find some new things from time to time at many shops. Individuals consign the clothing you will find and if the clothing sells, the profit is split between the store and the owner of the clothing. The new clothing that you will see comes from a number of sources. Some are from individuals that have just never worn an item and some comes from designers, manufacturers or retail establishments' overstock.

You will usually find a better quality of used clothing at these stores, as most are very selective in what they accept. The prices range anywhere from 30% of the retail value down to almost nothing. There are usually sale racks and some stores have a structured system for markdowns, such as 20% off after 30 days, 50% after 60 days, etc. Every consignment shop I have ever been to have end of season clearance sales, usually in January and August. The prices go way, way down and you can really get incredible deals at these times. Many stores will take requests, so if you have a favorite designer, let the owner know and you will be contacted when it becomes available.

Whenever you buy used clothing it is wise to check it over very carefully for any imperfections. Look closely for any stains, loose seams or tears that you may missed while trying it on. Consignment shops generally do not accept returns or exchanges of any kind, so know what you are buying before you buy it.

If you are looking to bring your clothes in to a consignment shop for consideration, there are a few things to remember. Make sure they are freshly cleaned and pressed and not more than a few seasons old. It is good to visit the store first to see what type of stock they carry. Some will want only couture and top designers while others will take any type of quality clothing as long as it is not too old. Talk to the owner to see what they are looking for. As I said before, they are very picky about what they accept, so don't waste your time or theirs. The split is usually 50/50 of the selling price and each store has their own methods of payment to the consignors.

Thrift shops are run mostly by not-for-profit organizations and the proceeds benefit these organizations, however there are exceptions to this rule. Prices are generally lower than the consignment shops and you will usually find more than clothing available. Some will also carry furniture, housewares, home décor, books, electronics and so on. These stores may not be as attractive as the consignment shops, but items can be priced so low it will send chills up your spine. I recently bought a $150 Rena Rowan summer dress for $8 at one. There are some thrift shops that you will find designer and brand name clothing on a very regular basis and others that are just hit and miss. Don't discount the latter entirely though, because those are the very ones where you may bag the most incredible bargains.

Long Island

Nassau – North Shore

Great Neck

National Council of Jewish Women Thrift Shop
587 Middle Neck Rd.
516-482-9246

M-F 10-4

This shop is chock full of clothing for the entire family, although they cater mostly to women. There are also a bit of small furniture and home décor items. In the boutique section you will find many of the top designers and there are lots of regular designer numbers and brand name items scattered throughout the rest of the store. Dresses and jackets start at $10 and blouses and slacks start at $5. A Tahari suit can go for $20, North Beach leather for $60 and Escada or Armani for $125. I also saw Liz Claiborne, Jones NY, Burberry and Carolyn Rhoem the last time I was there.

Hadassah Thrift Shop
734 Middle Neck Rd.
516-482-9246

Sun-Fri. 10-5

This shop is similar to a permanent rummage sale. You'll find clothing and housewares here and dedicated bargain hunters may come across a designer label or two. There are lots and lots of merchandise to pore through and prices are very reasonable. Dresses and jackets can start at $10, blouses $2 and slacks $3.

All Saint's Thrift
741 Middle Neck Rd.
516-482-9246

M-Sat. 10-4

This shop carries women, men and children's clothing, shoes, accessories, jewelry and some housewares. You will find designer and brand name labels here at good prices. Dresses go for $15-$100 for a top designer, jackets $15-$60, sweaters $8 and up and pants $10-$15. The last time I visited this store I saw a Tahari dress for $27, Evan Picone for $30 and Kenar for $20 a Georgio St. Angelo jacket for was marked $15 and an Oleg Casini suit $45. There were also some Liz Claiborne, Harve Bernard and Talbot's.

Checks are accepted.

Port Washington
St. Francis Thrift Shop
157 Main St
516-944-9090

Tues. & Thurs. 10-3
Wed. & Fri. 10-4
Sat. 10-2

This shop carries men, women and children's clothing, household items, books and more. They have a boutique section for their designer and brand name clothing. You may find a Kasper suit or Dior dress there from time to time. Dresses go for $10-$70, suits $20-$40, and blouses $2-$10. The proceeds go to St. Francis Hospital and you can bring in donations at any time.

JDRF Thrift Shop
93 Main St.
516-944-3623

M-F 10-4
Sat. 11-3 (call first to make sure they are open)

This store stocks women's clothing and they have lots of designer and brand names at very, very good prices. I've seen Christian Dior, Hanae Mori, Liz Claiborne and Dana Buchman suits for $15; Talbot's jackets for $8, and an Ellen Tracy outfit for $30. There were two pairs of Monolo

Blahnik shoes for $20 and a Karl Lagerfeld scarf for $3. I myself got a great Rena Rowan summer dress for $8 the last time I was there. This store benefits the Juvenile Diabetes Research Foundation and they accept donations at any time.

Checks are accepted.

St. Stephen's Church Consignment Shop
9 Carlton Ave.
516-944-8829

T, Th, Sat. 10-4
Closed July & August

You'll find clothing, shoes accessories, jewelry, housewares and home décor items in this shop. Prices are very, very reasonable and lots of designer names are available.

Checks are accepted.

Treasure Chest – Salvation Army
191 Main St.

M-F 10-4
Sat. 11-3

Women's, men and children's clothing, housewares, home décor.

Time & Again Family Consignment
101 Manorhaven Blvd.
516-883-6067

M-Sat. 11:30-5:30

This is a very nice consignment shop that has clothing for the whole family. Leave yourself lots of time to go through the racks here, because there is an enormous amount of merchandise to see and you don't want to miss anything. In addition to all the regular clothing you'll find bridal gowns, mother of the bride, vintage and a section of plus sizes. Prices are very reasonable with dresses averaging between $15-$25, slacks $9-$15, sweaters $8-$15 and jackets $15-$18. When I last visited this shop I saw a DKNY suit for $45, a Tahari dress for $35, a Talbot's linen dress for $12 and a Albert Nipon summer suit for $55. CeCe, the owner and all those who work here are very friendly and helpful to their customers, making it a very pleasant shopping experience. Consignments are accepted M-F from 12-4.

Checks are accepted.

Manhasset

The Corner Shop (Consignment)
593 Plandome Rd.
516-627-2883

M-T 1-4
W-Sat. 10-4

This store is unique in that it is a non-profit consignment shop. They do get very upscale merchandise including clothing, accessories, shoes, jewelry and giftware. Some of the designers you will find on a fairly regular basis are Chanel, Valentino, Dior, Donna Karan, and Ralph Lauren. Suits range from $28-$200, sweaters $10-30 and blouses $8-$24. The proceeds from this shop go to North Shore Child Guidance and they accept consignments by appointment only. You can bring in donations at any time.

Checks are accepted.

Glen Cove

Fabulous Finds (Consignment)
12 School St.
516-759-6870

Tues. – Sat. 10-5

This is another great consignment shop stocked with lots of designer and brand name women's clothing, handbags, shoes, accessories and jewelry. You'll find Escada, St. John, Prada, Gucci and Vera Wang. Dresses range from $16-$18, suits $18-$100, suits $21-$200, blouses and slacks $10 and up. They use a structured markdown system with prices knocked down 50% after 30 days. After 60 days leftovers are donated to local charities. The handbags and shoes are all top quality designer names also. Consignments are accepted T-Sat. 10-2 by appointment only

All major credit cards are accepted.

Family & Children's Thrift
190 Glen Cove Rd. (Sea Cliff Ave.)
516-671-7929

M-Th 10-5
F 10-5:30
Sat. 10-5
Sun. 12-4

You'll find women's, men's and children's clothing, shoes and linens. There is a designer rack and prices are good. This shop benefits the Family & Children's Association and they accept donations at any time.

Checks are accepted

Locust Valley
Again & Again (Consignment)
296 Forest Ave.
516-674-6180

M-Sat. 11-6

This shop carries women and children's clothing and home décor. You'll find a decent amount of designer names available among the merchandise. I've seen Ralph Lauren, Ann Klein, Cacharel and Ann Taylor to name a few. There are also some very interesting items for the home. Consignments are accepted by appointment only.

Oyster Bay
Next to New Boutique (Consignment)
59 W. Main St.
516-922-2880

M-Sat. 10-5

This boutique carries women's clothing, accessories, shoes and jewelry. It's a very nice little store with names like St. John, Chanel, Armani, Donna Karan and Kamali passing through on a regular basis along with a long list of other more moderately priced lines. Prices are reasonable with dresses selling for $18-$21, slacks $16-$18, blouses $12-$14 and jackets $24 and up. Please make an appointment to bring in consignments.

Major credit cards are accepted.

Bayville

Selective Boutique (Consignment)

259 Bayville Ave. (Shore Rd)
516-922-2680

Tues.-Sat. 10-6
Sun. 11-6

This shop, which is a little off the beaten track in Bayville, is a definite find. Lots of great women's clothing, shoes, handbags and jewelry can be had here for very good prices. There are also new, quite unique gift items imported from Italy available. You'll find lots of designer and brand name labels such as Jones NY, ABS, Ann Klein, Harve Bernard, St. John and Chanel. After 5 dresses can range from $26-$80, slacks $10-$25, and casual dresses from $20 and up. Consignments are taken by appointment only.

Major credit cards are accepted.

Nassau – Mid Island

Hempstead

Josie's Thrift Shop

113 Fulton Ave.
516-292-6267

M-Th. 10-6
Fri. 10-7
Sun. 12-5

This store features men, women's and children's clothing. You will find some designer names here and prices are very reasonable. Dresses range from $1-$25, slacks $1-$4, and suits from $5-$70

Major credit cards are accepted.

Mercy Medical Center Thrift Shop
369 Peninsula Blvd.
516-481-9379

M-Sat. 10-3

You'll find women's, men's and children's clothing, bric-a-brac and small appliances at this shop. There are some designer and brand names to be had here, such as Kasper, Jones NY, Evan Picone and Larry Levine. Dresses are $10, slacks $4, jackets $5 and blouses $3.

East Meadow
Veronica's Closet (Children's Consignment0
391 Merrick Ave.
516-483-4764

M-Sat. 10-5

This store carries children's clothing, women's handbags, sunglasses and accessories. Please make an appointment to bring in consignments.

Westbury
St. Brigid's Attic (Thrift)
178 Post Ave.
516-876-0252

M-Sat. 10-3

Women's, men's and children's clothing and household items can be found here. Dresses are $10, jackets $5, blouses $2, slacks $2 and up and men's suits $5.

Levittown
Salvation Army Thrift Store
148 Gardiners Ave.
516-731-9631

M-Sat. 9-5
Clothing, furniture, household items, books and electronics.

MC and Visa are accepted.

Farmingdale

New To You Shop (Thrift)
401 Main St.
516-752-2181

W-Sat. 10-3:30

This store has women's, men's and children's clothing, antiques, books, toys and housewares. There is a boutique section featuring better women's items.

Pretty New Shop (Thrift)
187 Main St.
516-420-1394

M-Sat. 10-4

You'll find men's, women's and children's clothing and housewares at this store. Clothing is mainly middle of the road, but you will come across an occasional designer label. Dresses are $6-$10, jackets $5-%6, slacks and blouses $3.

St. Sarkis Thrift Store
301 Main St.
516-756-5171

M-Sat. 9:30-6
Sun. 11-3

This store carries clothing, bric-a-brac and odds and ends. I found lots of designer suits priced, God bless them, sinfully low. Kasper, Harve Bernard, Liz Claiborne, Cache and Georgio St. Angelo were some of them all going for $10-$15. Dresses go for $8 and up, jackets $5 and up, blouses $2 and up and slacks $2-$6.

MC, Visa and Amex accepted.

Hicksville
Mickie & Co. (Consignment)
15 W. Nicholai St.
516-942-5572

M-Sat. 11:30-4:30
Closed Wed.

Approximately 25% of this store features clothing. The rest is comprised of nick knacks, fabric, furniture, housewares, and home décor and you can find some unusual items here. Consignments are accepted by appointment only.

Nassau – South Shore

East Rockaway
Carmela Thrift Fair
31 Main St.
516-593-2338

M-Sat. 10-4

This store features men, women's and children's clothing, handbags, jewelry, housewares and nick knacks. This is a good amount of designer and brand name labels available. Slacks, dresses, blouses and skirts range from $6-$20.

Checks are accepted.

Oceanside
Cooky's Thrift & Consignment
224 Merrick Rd.
516-766-1436

M-Sat. 10-5
Sun. 12-5

You'll find men's and women's clothing, furniture, and bric-a-brac at this shop. There are some designer items to be had, such as Donna Karan, Chanel and Prada.

Checks are accepted.

Hewlett
The Emperor's Old Clothes
300 Mill Rd. (W. Bdwy)
516-569-2639

M-Th. 11-4
Or by appointment

This shop carries top designers only -Chanel, Hermes, Gucci, Fendi, Prada, Dolce & Gabanna- to name a few. It is not a storefront, it's in an office building and try-ons are permitted. Some recent finds include a Chanel suit for $800, Ungaro blazer for $45, Escada silk blouse for $50, or Rena Lange sweater for $50. They do have men's accessories also. Grab a Hermes tie for your man at a mere $25. They also sell on Ebay, in fact that is where they got their start. Their ID is z.emperors.old.clothes or you can email them at sales@theemperorsoldclothes.com.

Valley Stream

Community Presbyterian Thrift
409 Rockaway Ave.
516-561-8543

M-Sat. 11:30-3:30
Closed Thurs.

This store carries women's, men's and children's clothing, housewares and bric-a-brac. Slacks and blouses are $3, dresses and jackets run from $5-$10.

Franklin Hospital Medical Center Thrift Shop
138 Rockaway Ave.
516-825-5216

M-Sat. 10-4

You can get women, men and children's clothing, furniture, housewares, bric-a-brac, linens and more at this store. There is a decent amount of upscale clothing to be found here, with names like Harve Bernard and Liz Claiborne among them. Dresses range from $10-$80, slacks $5-$30, jackets $10-$60 and blouses $5-$50.

Visa and MC are accepted.

Alba's Thrift Shop
4 E. Valley Stream Blvd.
516-561-6901

M-Sat. 10-6

Men's, women and children's clothing can be found here at very low prices. Most items range from $1-$5.

Freeport

Mana Thrift Store
575 Main St.
516-623-4310

M-Sat. 10:30-7
Sun. 1-6

This store carries men's, women's and children's clothing, housewares and furniture. They do get designer and brand name labels such as Calvin Klein, Ann Taylor and Christian Dior. Prices are low, so there's a good chance to nab a real bargain here. Jeans and dresses start at $2.50, blouses and slacks at $1.99.

Bellmore

Elite Repeat Boutique (Consignment)
2920 Merrick Rd.
516-785-2903

Th-Sat 11:30-5

You could literally spend half the day poring through all the clothing in this store. It is jam packed with women's clothing, accessories, handbags, shoes and jewelry. You will find lots of designer and brand names here, with Ralph Lauren, Ann Klein, Dana Buchman, Prada, and Chanel among them. There is also a large selection of sizes 18-24 and Gerry, the owner, gets in new designer perfumes and eyeglass frames on a regular basis. Dresses range from $18-$110, pants $10-$28, After 5 $30-$200, jackets $18-$48 and furs $80-$1000.

Checks accepted.

Seaford

Open Door Thrift Shop
2142 Jackson Ave.
516-221-2222

M-Sat. 10-4

This is your typical all around thrift shop with clothing for the family, bric-a-brac, books and odd and ends. The prices are very reasonable and you can find some very nice pieces of clothing here. The store benefits the Central Nassau Guidance Center.

Massapequa

St. Rose of Lima Community Thrift Shop
4318 Merrick Rd.
516-799-5212

M-Th 10-3

This store carries mostly clothing for the whole family with a small amount of housewares thrown in. Prices are low, ranging from $3-$7 for most items. Some designer names do pass through here from time to time.

Western Suffolk– North Shore

Huntington
Confidence Closet (Thrift)
1805 New York Ave. (West Hills Rd.)
631-424-7848

W-F 11-3
Sat. 11-4
Sun. 11-5

This shop carries women's and children's clothing, accessories, shoes, jewelry and bric-a-brac. There are quite a bit of designer and brand name labels passing through here on a regular basis and prices are very reasonable. Dresses start at $6, pants $4, jackets $6, blouses $2 and suits $13. You find Jones NY, Donna Karan and ABS to name a few. The proceeds from this store benefit a domestic abuse service agency and those women who are trying to escape the cycle of violence and re-enter the work force can come here to be outfitted at no charge. Donations are accepted Thursday and Saturday.

Checks are accepted.

North Shore Holiday House (Thrift)
74 Huntington Rd.
631-427-2944

T-Sat. 10—4
Closed from Memorial Day to Labor Day

This store, which is tucked away from the shopping district on a beautiful tree lined road, is a great find. You'll find clothes for the whole family, furniture, bric-a-brac, housewares, toys and books. I've seen dresses by Jones NY, Harve Bernard, Evan Picone, Tahari, August Silk and LL Bean for $8: Ann Taylor jackets for $8, slacks for $6 and suits for $12. Most of the clothing here is designer or brand name and they also have a $1 room. This store benefits the Holiday House camp for underprivileged girls and is housed on its grounds, hence the summer closing. In the weeks before they close on Memorial Day prices are marked down 50% and in the last days everything is $1. Donations are accepted T-F 10-4 and Sat. 10-1.

Checks are accepted.

Community Thrift Shop
8 E. Carver St.
631-241-4883

M-Sat.
10-4

This is a large shop that offers men's, women's
and children's clothing, accessories, shoes,
jewelry, housewares, home décor and books. You
will find some designer and brand name clothing
here and they have a boutique section, which holds
the After 5 items. Prices are very reasonable with
most things priced at $1-$40. The proceeds from
this store benefits many charities and you can
bring in your donations at any time.

St. Patrick's Trocaire Thrift Shop
630 New York Ave.
631-673-5328

M-F 9-4
Sat. 10-1

This shop carries men's, women's and children's
clothing, housewares and toys. You'll find lots of
designer and brand name items, including Eddie
Bauer, Ann Taylor, Express, Gap, Old Navy,
Calvin Klein and Liz Claiborne. There is also a
boutique rack with higher end and After 5
numbers. Dresses range from $5-$8, suits $8 and
blouses and slacks $3. This shop benefits St.
Patrick's Human Services and clothing is provided

free of charge to those who qualify. Donations are accepted M-F 9-3 and Sat. 10-1.

Greenlawn

Penny Wise Thrift Shop
54 Bdwy
631-261-0477

M-Sat. 12-8

In this store you will find clothing, mostly women's and general thrift shop merchandise. Dresses range $12-$60, jackets $12-$40, slacks $6-$15 and sweaters $5-$65.

Checks are accepted.

Northport

St. Paul's Thrift Shop
284 Main St.
631-262-9167

T, F, & Sat. 10-3:30

You'll find clothing for the entire family here at very low prices. Dresses range from $3-$4, slacks $3.50 and blazers $3.50.

Cow Harbor Kids (Thrift)
491 Main St.
631-757-6568

M-Sat. 10-4
W & Th. till 5

This store carries children's clothing and equipment and maternity wear. You will find brand and designer names here, such as Guess and Calvin Klein. Clothing ranges from $2-$15. This store benefits the United Way and donations are accepted any day until one hour before closing. Please call ahead to donate.

Checks are accepted.

Western Suffolk – Mid Island

East Northport
Act II Consignment Boutique
248 Larkfield Rd.
(Moving to 11 Hewitt Sq., Larkfield & Pulaski Rd., in June, 2002)
631-754-1800

M-F 10-6
Th. till 8
Sat. 10-5

Just about all of the women's clothing, shoes and handbags in this store are designer and brand name. The prices are usually 1/3 of the original retail value or less. Some of the things I have seen here are an Ann Taylor twin set at $29, a BCBG blouse at $16, an Escada sweater set at $59, and a Chanel silk jacket at $150. The last time I visited this store there was a new with tag $200 Fal cashmere sweater for $39 and a $600 Philippe Adec $600 pantsuit for $98. Many high-end handbags such as Prada, Kate Spade, Coach and Fendi are here on a regular basis. The markdowns are taken in a structured manner, will the prices going down 20% after 30 days and $50 after 60. Look for their clearance sales in January and August with prices up to 80% off the original.

MC, Visa, Amex, and checks are accepted.

Salvation Army Thrift Store
319 Clay Pitts Rd.
631-368-1170

M-F 10-3
Sat. 10-2

Clothing and housewares.

Major credit cards are accepted.

Goodwill Thrift Store
1900 E. Jericho Tpk.
631-462-4219

M-Sat. 9:30-8
Sun. 11-6
This store carries clothing for the whole family, furniture, housewares, toys and electronics. There is quite a bit of designer and brand names scattered throughout the racks and the prices are low, low, low. It's definitely worth the trip.

Major credit cards accepted.

Nesconset

Ali's Closet (Consignment)
215 Smithtown Blvd.
631-360-8757

M-T-W 10-5
Th. 11-7
F-Sat. 11-5

You'll find women's clothing, shoes, accessories, handbags and jewelry at this shop. Many designer and brand name labels pass through here on a regular basis. Some of the clothes that have been found here are Donna Karan, Michael Kors, Ellen

Tracy and Jones NY. Dresses range from $12-$15, slacks $8-$15, blouses $5-$10 and jackets $15.

Visa, Amex, MC, Discover is accepted.

Ronkonkoma

Nearly New Shop (Thrift)
15 E. Lake Terrace
631-588-2057

M-W-Th.-Sat. 11-4

You'll find clothing, housewares and bric-a-brac at this shop. The proceeds benefit St. Mary's Episcopal Church and donations are accepted at any time.

Options for Community Living Thrift Shop
392 Hawkins Ave.
631-981-7626

T-Sat. 10-4

You'll find clothing for the whole family along with household items at this store. Prices range from $3-$8 and you can find some designer and brand names here.

J&C Thrift Store
2411 Chestnut Ave.
631-467-2071

M-Sat. 10-5

There is clothing for the family here, including wedding gowns, tuxedos and leather goods. Prices range from $1.99-$150. You can find some designer and brand name clothing here. Credit cards are accepted.

Western Suffolk – South Shore

Amityville
Church Attic Thrift Shop
47 Bdwy
631-264-4555

M-F 10-4

This store carries clothing and household items. You will find some designer names such as Liz Claiborne and Jones NY, however most are the mid-priced lines. Dresses range $5-$25, jackets $5-$15, blouses $2-$4 and slacks $3.

Cloak Room Thrift Shop
227 Bdwy
631-598-1134

M-Sat. 10-3:45

This shop has men's, women's and children's clothing, housewares, bric-a-brac and toys. Dresses ranges $4-$15, pants $1-$5 and tops $2-$5. Proceeds benefit St. Martin of Tours.

Georgia's Bargains on Broadway
232 Bdwy
631-789-9736

T-Sat. 10-3

You will find mainly odds and ends in this shop, however there is one small rack of clothing to look through and I must say I did find designer names among them.

Babylon
St. Joseph's Thrift Shop
34 Grove Pl.
631-669-5574

M-W-Th. 10-3

This is a typical church thrift store stocking clothes for the family, housewares, furniture and bric-a-brac. There is quite a lot of clothing to choose from and you may run into a designer name or two.

Good Samaritan Thrift Shop
179 Deer Park Ave.
631-376-3499

M-Sat. 10-4

This shop carries clothing for the family, household items, bric-a-brac, books, toys and games. The clothing is of good quality with many designer and brand names passing through on a regular basis. Prices are also very reasonable, ranging from $2-$20 for most items. They have 50% off sales on a regular basis.

Bon Marché (Thrift)
45 E. Main St.
631-321-5945

T-Sat. 10-4

You will find a large assortment of women's clothing, accessories and shoes at this shop.

Bay Shore

Pandora's Box (Thrift)
94 W. Main St.
631-968-7317

M 10-2
T-F 10-4
Sat. 10-3

There are men, women's and children's clothing to
be found at this store along with furniture
housewares and appliances. Prices for clothing are
quite low ranging from $2-$5.

St. Peter's Thrift Shop
150 S. Country Rd.
631-206-1091

T & Sat 11-3

This shop has clothing for the family, housewares
and bric-a-brac. Prices range from $1-$5

Islip

St. Mary's Church Thrift Shop
585 Main St.
631-581-7666

M-Sat. 10-3:45

You'll find clothes for the family, toys and odds &
ends here. Prices for clothing range from $2-$15

Eastern Suffolk-North Shore

Port Jefferson

St. Charles Consignment Shop
427 Myrtle Ave.
631-474-6866

T & Sat. 10-2
W-F 11-3

This shop carries clothing, jewelry and bric-a-brac.
You'll find a bit of designer and brand names
scattered throughout. Dresses range from $4-$15,
slacks $3-$10, jackets $10 and blouses $3.

PJ's Second Time Around (Thrift)
1518 Main St.
631-331-1276

M-Sat. 12-5

You'll find women's, men's and children's
clothing, small furniture and bric-a-brac in this
shop. Dresses range from $4-$10, jackets $5-$10,

pants $2-$5 and blouses from $3-$5. You many find some designer clothing here.

Stony Brook

Anew Boutique (Consignment)
2194 Nesconset Hwy. (Waldbaum's shopping center)
631-751-5111

M-Sat. 10-6
Sun. 12-5

This shop has women's clothing, accessories, shoes, handbags and jewelry. You will find designer and brand name apparel here. Carol Little, Ann Taylor, and Tahari are some that I have seen here. Prices range anywhere from $2-$100 and there is quite a large section of plus sizes.

Credit cards and checks are accepted.

Riverhead

Salvation Army
319 E. Main St.
631-727-1571

M-Sat. 9-4:50

Clothing, furniture, housewares, appliances.

Eastern Suffolk – South Shore

Bellport
Bellport Methodist Thrift Shop
185 S. Country Rd.
631-286-0746

T-Sat. 10-4

This store carries men's, women's and children's clothing, furniture, housewares, and books. There are lots of designer and brand names to be found here. Liz Claiborne, Bergdorf Goodman, Evan Picone, Gap, and Banana Republic are some of them. Prices are very low, so you can practically steal some of these great items. Dresses are $3-$5, jackets $5, blouses, skirts, slacks and jeans are $.75 and sweaters are 2/$1.

Sayville
St. Lawrence Thrift Shop
111 Railroad Ave.
631-567-1592

M-Sat. 10-3:30

You'll find clothing for the whole family and bric-a-brac at this shop. Liz Claiborne, Sag Harbor and London Fog are some of the recognizable names you will see here. Dresses and jackets are $4 and up, slacks and blouses $2.50 and up.

Noah's Ark Thrift Shop
245 Main St.
631-218-9454

M-F 11-5
W 11-8
Sun. 11-5

You'll find clothing for the family, housewares and toys in this shop. Prices range from $2-$12 for the clothing.

Checks are accepted.

Center Moriches

Moriches Bay Historical Society (Consignment & Thrift)
23 Montauk Hwy.
631-878-1776

Sat. 10-5

This shop has a small amount of clothing along with furniture and housewares.

Westhampton

St. Mark's Store (Thrift)
Main St. (on church grounds)
631-288-2628

W-F 10-3
Sat. 10-1

There is women's, men's and children's clothing, furniture and housewares at this store. You will find many designer and brand name here. Prices start at $4 and go up.

Checks are accepted.

East End Hospice Thrift Shop
58 Riverhead Rd.
631-288-3268

Th-Sat. 10-4

You'll find women's, men's and children's clothing, accessories, jewelry and furniture here. Much of the clothes are high-end designer and brand name. Prices from $1-$50.

Checks are accepted.

E Quoge

Once Upon a Time
489 Montauk Hwy.
631-653-8197

M-Th & Sat 10-5
F 10-6
Sun. 12-4

This store carries women's clothing, shoes, accessories and jewelry. It is the only consignment clothing shop on the East End and it is full of great items. Lots of designers like Donna Karan, Jones NY, Liz Claiborne and more can be found at very reasonable prices. It's right on the highway and worth the stop on your way to weekend fun in the sun.

Sag Harbor

Dominican Sisters Thrift Shop
Washington St.
631-725-0861

M-Sat. 10-4

This store carries clothing for the whole family, housewares and books. You can find designer and brand names on a consistent basis. Slacks and shirts are $4 and up. Dresses start at $7.50, coats $10, blazers $8 and blouses $3.

Southampton

Discovery Shop (Thrift)

22 Nugent St.
631-283-6789

M-Sat. 10-4

This is an American Cancer Society thrift shop, which are known for their designer and brand name clothing. You'll also find furniture, bric-a-brac and books here. Dresses range from $10-$30, blouses $5-$30, jackets $8-30 and slacks $5-$25.

Birthright of Peconic Thrift Shop

17 Flying Point Rd.
631-287-6456

M-Sat. 11-3

This shop has men's, women's and children's clothing, housewares and bric-a-brac. On Saturdays you will also find furniture. They have a lot of designer and new clothing coming in on a regular basis, especially new children's clothes. Dresses and slacks start at $5, jackets $8 and blouses $3.

Water Mill

Animal Rescue Fund Thrift Shop
670 Montauk Hwy.
631-726-6613

M-Sat. 10-3:45
Closed Wed. during off-season.
Sun. 11-3

This store has clothing for the family, furniture, bric-a-brac, home décor and books. The clothing is of a very good quality with many designer and brand names to be found. There is also a boutique section with wedding gowns, tuxedos and new items. Sweaters, skirts and slacks start at $5 and go up. Dresses start at $8 and t-shirts $1.50

Bridgehampton

St. Ann's Thrift Shop
2463 Main St.
631-537-5150

F-Sat. 10-4

You'll find men's, women's and children's clothing, small furniture and bric-a-brac here. There is also a designer boutique section carrying the better items. Prices go from $4-$10.

East Hampton

Animal Rescue Fund Thrift Shop
458 Pantigo Rd.
631-324-9370

M-Sun. 10-3:30

See listing above.

Eastern Suffolk – Mid Island

Medford

St. Sylvester's Thrift Shop
69 Ohio Ave
631-475-3076

T & Th. 10-3
Wed. 10-3 & 5:30-7:30
Sat. 10-1

At this shop clothing is sold by the pound, ranging from $1-$2 per.   You'll find men's, women's and children's and housewares.

Be Pennywise
2289 Rt. #112
631-475-3076

M-Sat. 10:30-6
Sun. 10:30-4

This is an ongoing, indoor yard sale. You'll find a little bit of everything from clothing to CDs to housewares and everything in between. Prices are very low, starting at a mere $.25.

Manhattan

Below Houston

Church St. Surplus (Thrift)
327 Church St. (Canal & Lipsenard)
212-226-5280

M-Sat. 10:30-6

This is a retail store of used clothing, both men's and women's. They buy their merchandise outright from distributors.

MC, Visa, Discover are accepted.

New & Almost New (Consignment)
65 Mercer St. (Spring & Broome)
212-226-6677

M-F 12-6:30
Sat. 1-6

Contemporary designer clothing is the mainstay of this shop with a small amount of vintage available too. MiuMiu, Yohij, Yamonamoto, Chanel, Dolce & Gabanna, and Gucci are some of the labels that pass through on a regular basis. This store caters

to sizes small to medium, as many model consign
their castoffs here. Dresses range from $45-$200,
suits can go up to $200 for an Armani, blouses,
start at $25 and there is a great $9 box.
Consignments are accepted weekdays by
appointment only.

Visa, MC, Amex, Discover, JCB are accepted.

Salvation Army
115 Allen St. (Delancy)
212-2542816

M-Sat. 10-5:45

Clothing, Furniture, Housewares, Electronics.

East Side
Houston – 14th

Good Old Lower East Side (Thrift)
17 Avenue B   (2nd St.)
212-358-1041

M-Thurs. 10-6
F & Sat. 11-8

Women's, men's and children's clothing, jewelry
and houswares are available here. A large amount
of the clothing has recognizable labels, ranging

from the Gap to Chanel. Prices are very
reasonable. Women's dresses and slacks go for
$8-$12, suits for $15-$20. Men's shirts are $8-$12
and suits $20-$30. This store benefits the
Community Housing Project and donations are
accepted anytime.

Visa, MC, Discover are accepted.

Tokio 7 (Consignment)
64 E. 7th St. (1st & 2nd)
212-353-8443

M-Sun. 12-8:30

This store carries upscale designer clothing for the
young, trendy crowd. Prada, Gucci and YSL are
just some of the names you'll see here and there is
a wide range of prices. You can get things for
anywhere to $2-$400. They request that you make
an appointment if you have more then 10 items for
consignment.

Visa, MC, Amex is accepted.

West Side
Houston – 14th

St. Luke's Thrift Shop
487 Hudson St. (Grove)
212-924-9364

M-F 11-6
Thurs. till 7
Sat. 10-6

You will find women's, men's and children's clothing here along with shoes, accessories, bric-a-brac, books and china. Approximately 30% of the clothing has designer labels, such as Donna Karan, Armani, Hugo Boss, Josie Natori, Chanel, and Dior. The prices are reasonable. Dresses go for $12-$15, with designer numbers going for $50-$75. Slacks are $7-$25, suits $25-$40 and blouses $6-$15. This proceeds of this store benefit St. Luke's outreach programs and you can bring in your donations M-F 11-3 and Sat. 10-1. Please limit them to 3 large shopping bags.

Visa, MC, Amex and accepted.

East Side
14th – 59th

St. George's Thrift Shop
61 Gramercy Park N. (Park & Lexington)
212-475-2674

M-F 10:30-5:30
Sat. 10:30-4

An assortment of clothing, jewelry, housewares, furniture and bric-a-brac will be found here. Dresses range from $6-$10, slacks $6-$8, suits $10-$25 and blouses $4-$6. There is a small men's and children's area with men's suits going for $15-$20. This store benefits St. George's outreach programs and they accept donations at any time.

MC, Visa, Amex, Checks are accepted.

Vintage Thrift Store
286 3rd Ave. (22nd & 23rd)
212-871-0777

M-Thurs. 10:30-8
F 10:30 – Dusk
Sat. Closed
Sun. 11-7

This shop carries women's and men's clothing, jewelry, housewares, furniture, and bric-a-brac. About 10% of the clothing are designer names with Geoffrey Beene, Armani, and vintage Halston making appearances. Women's dresses range from $20-$50, slacks $10-$30, suits $30-$75 and blouses $10-$25. Men's suits range from $45-$75

All major credit cards are accepted.

Housing Works (Thrift)
157 E. 23rd St. (Lex. & 3rd)
212-529-5955

M-Sat. 10-6
Sun. 12-5

This is a fabulous thrift shop that carries clothing, furniture and home décor. You'll find lots of designer and brand names at great prices.

Major credit cards accepted.

City Opera Thrift Shop
222 E. 23rd St. (2nd & 3rd)
212-684-5344

M-Sat. 10-6
Sun. 12-5

You will find women's and men's clothing here along with furniture, bric-a-brac, home décor, rugs, fabric and records. Some of the furniture is antique as well as the clothing vintage. About 15% of the clothing is designer with Donna Karan, Mark Montano, and Ralph Lauren passing through. Prices are good, with slacks going for $5-$30, dresses $5-$300 with those at the $300 end being a Chanel leather number or the like. Suits go for $25-$35 and blouses at around $10. Proceeds from this store benefit the NYC Opera and donations are accepted anytime.

All major credit cards and travelers checks are accepted.

Salvation Army Thrift Store
220 E. 23rd St. (2nd & 3rd)
212-532-8115

M-F 10-7:15
Sat. 10-6

Clothing, furniture, housewares, toys, bric-a-brac, electronics.

Faith, Hope & Charity Thrift Shop
402 3rd Ave. (28th & 29th)
212-725-4721

M-Sat. 11-8
Sun. 11-7

Women's and men's clothing, housewares, computers, stereos, CDs and shoes can all be found here. About 75% of the women's clothing is designer with Ann Taylor, Harve Bernard, Ellen Tracy, Dior, Kasper and Armani included. They have a special boutique section with high-end designer duds. Dresses range from $6-$25, slacks $6-$15, suits $25-$45 and blouses $2-$12. This store benefits the St. Union Deliverance Church and accepts donations anytime.

Visa, MC, Discover are accepted.

Helpline Thrift Shop
382 3rd Ave. (29th)
212-532-5136

M-Sat. 10:30-7:30
Sun. 12-5

They carry women's, men's and children's clothing, jewelry, bric-a-brac, and furniture. They also have lots of new things at this store. About 35% of the store is clothing, with 50% of that being designer. Some that have been there are Perry Ellis, Barney's, Ann Taylor, and Ann Klein. Dresses range from $5-$15, slacks $2-$40 and suits from$5-$50. This store benefits the Helpline Telephone services and they will accept donations anytime.

Visa, MC and Checks are accepted.

Exchange Unlimited (Consignment)
563 2nd Ave. (31st St.)
212-889-3229

This consignment shop carries women and men's clothing with approximately 25%-40% being designer labels. Ralph Lauren and Ferragamo are a couple of the many that pass through there. Women's dresses, slacks and suits range from $8-$20 and men's suits from $10-$50. They accept consignments by appointment only.

Checks are accepted.

West Side
14th – 59th

Rags a Gogo (Thrift)
218 W. 14th St. (7th & 8th)
646-486-4011

M-Sat. 11-8
Sun. 12-7

This store carries casual second hand clothes. You will find jeans, t-shirts, hoodies, track, denim, a small selection of dresses and leather jackets & boots and. Everything is $25 or below.

All major credit cards are accepted.

Housing Works (Thrift)
143 W. 17th St. (6th & 7th)
212-366-0820

M-Sat. 10-6
Sun. 12-5

This is a fabulous thrift shop that carries clothing, furniture and home décor. You'll find lots of designer and brand names at great prices.

Major credit cards accepted.

Fisch for the Hip (Consignment)
(Formerly Out of Our Closet)
15 W. 18th St. (6th & 7th)
212-633-9053

M-Sat. 12-7
Sun. 12-6

Upscale women's and men's clothing are the order of the day here and you will find the likes of

Chanel, Dolce & Gabanna, Prada, Hermes and Gucci on a regular basis. Dresses start at $150, suits $100-$600, slacks $50-$150 and blouses $60-$400. Consignments are accepted anytime.

Visa, MC, Amex, JCB are accepted.

Angel Street Thrift Shop
118 W. 17th St.   (6th & 7th)
212-229-0546

M-Sat. 10-6
Sun. 12-5

This thrift shop carries women's, men's and children's clothing, furniture and household items. You will find lots of designer and brand name labels here. Calvin Klein, Donna Karan, Ralph Lauren, Isaac Mizrahi, and Burberry are just a few of them. Dresses and slacks start at $3 and go up and suits start at $5. This store benefits Lower East Side Services and they accept donations at any time. The also have a free pick-up service.

MC, Visa, Amex, Debit Cards are accepted.

Salvation Army Thrift Shop
208 8th Ave. (20th & 21st)
212-929-5214

M-F 10-7

Sat. 10-5:30

536 W. 46th St. (10th & 11th)
212-664-8563

M-Sat. 9:30-5:45

Clothing, furniture, housewares.

Outcasts (Thrift)
660 10th Ave. (47th)
212-974-0121

M-Sat. 10:30-6

You'll find women's and men's clothing,
housewares, bric-a-brac and books at this shop.
They do get quite a bit of designer and brand name
clothing in on a regular basis. Some of the names
you'll see are Chanel and Albert Nippon. Prices
range from $4-$100. The proceeds benefit St.
Clement's Episcopal Church and donations are
accepted at any time.

Ritz Furs (Consignment)
107 W. 57th St. (6th & 7th)
212-265-4559

M-Sat. 9-6
Closed Sat. July

Open Sun. 12-5 Nov.- Feb.

The Ritz has been offering pre-owned furs to NY for over 50 years. Their selection includes everything from mink, to fox, to sable, to lamb. Many of the top designer labels are found here along with a vintage and retro section. Mink coats which retail for $6000-$9000 can be had here for $2000-$3000. If you like Fox you can grab a jacket that was originally $3500 for $1000. They have fur-trimmed coats, jackets, gloves, headbands, bags and more. Sable can range from $2000-$20,000. At the time of printing they offered a free pair of mink earmuffs with every purchase, so be sure to inquire if they are still doing this.

Major credit cards are accepted.

East Side
59th - 96th

Margoth Consignment Shop
218 E. 81st St. (2nd & 3rd)
212-988-7688

M-Sat 11-7
Sun. 12-5

This is a brand new shop tucked away on 81st St. and it is a gem. This store is packed with all of the designers we love. You'll find Chanel, Hermes, Escada, Dolce & Gabanna, YSL, Dior, Vuitton, Tod's, Armani, Issey Miyake, and lots of Prada. Margoth gets new Chanel handbags, designer perfumes and shoes. Chanel starts at $125, Dolce & Gabanna at $75-$100, Escada $100-$150, a Gucci which retails for $400 at $125 here. There is really something for everyone here. Blouses start at $20 and dresses at $50. I nabbed the most beautiful silk bias cut dress here for just $50. Make this store a definite stop on you list. They accept consignments anytime and will take special requests from customers.

MC, Visa, Amex, and Travelers Checks are accepted.

Tatiana Designer Resale (Consignment)
767 Lexington Ave. (60th & 61st)
5th Floor
212-717-7684

M-F 11am-7pm
Sat. 11am-6pm

This is an upscale consignment shop carrying high-end contemporary women's and men's clothing, and vintage couture. They also have accessories and shoes. Some of the designers they carry are Gucci, Prada, Hermes, Fendi, and Chanel. Get an $800 pair of Dolce and Gabanna pants for $45, a brand new Roberto Cavalli showroom piece for $200 that would sell for $1000 retail. Chanel starts at $300 and goes up. Tatiana gets many new items from the top designer showrooms on a daily basis. She will accept consignments at any time and will also make house calls to pick them up in and around the city.

All major credit cards are accepted.

Housing Works (Thrift)
202 E.77th St. (2nd & 3rd)
212-772-8461

M-Sat. 10-6
Sun. 12-5

This is a fabulous thrift shop that carries clothing, furniture and home décor. You'll find lots of designer and brand names at great prices.

Major credit cards accepted.

La Boutique Resale (Consignment)
1045 Madison Ave. (79th & 80th)
2nd Floor
212-517-8099

M-Sat 11-6:30
Sun. 12-6

As one of the great Madison Avenue consignment shops, you can find Chanel, Armani, Prada, Gucci, St. John, Issey Miyake, Dolce and Gabanna, and on and on here regularly. There is a very nice vintage couture section featuring Halston, Pucci, Pauline Trigere and Courreges to name a few. Dresses start at about $50 and you can get a Chanel Suit that retails for $2600 and up here for $500 - $1200. The last time I was there, I saw a brand new Chanel Suit from the current season, tags still on for $1100. Escada jackets start at $60. And if you're in the market for something a little less pricey there are many things to choose form. They carry up to size 18. Jonathan accepts consignments anytime and he will pay cash on the spot for Chanel or St. John

All Major credit cards are accepted.

A Second Chance (Consignment)
1109 Lexington Ave. (77th & 78th)
212-744-6041
2nd Floor
M-F 11-7
Sat. 11-6

This consignment shop carries primarily designer clothing. The usual suspects –Hermes, Chanel, Prada, Gucci, Judith Leiber, Armani are found here. There is many, many Chanel items here and new designer shoes – Chanel, Prada, Tod's – come in on a regular basis. You'll pay $200 for a pair that retail for $400-$500. Slacks can range from $25 up to $200 for an $800 pair by Chanel. Dresses start at $45 and a $1000 Herve Leger number goes for $400. A lovely suit can be gotten for a mere $75, or you can go for the Chanel at $1000. A $2500 Armani suit can be stolen for $300. Blouses range from $25 - $200. Consignments are accepted anytime

Visa, MC, Amex is accepted.

Arthritis Foundation Thrift
121 E. 77th St. (Park and Lex)
212-772-8816

M – Sat. 10 – 5:45

This store is about 50% designer clothes. Hermes, Ungaro, YSL, Valentino, Chanel and Escada are frequent visitors, to name a few. Prices are quite reasonable. You can grab a pair of pants for $8 - $30, a dress for $10 - $25 with special couture numbers going for up to $1000, suits for $30 - $50 and blouses $10 - $20. They also have men's and children's clothing, bric-a-brac, jewelry and small furniture. The proceeds from this store go to the NY Chapter of the Arthritis Foundation. They accept donations anytime.

Visa, MC, Amex is accepted.

Michael's Consignment Shop for Women
1041 Madison Ave. (79th & 80th)
212-737-7273

M-Sat. 9:30-6
Thursday till 8pm
Closed Sat. and Sun. from July 4th to Labor Day

This is another one of those great Madison Avenue consignment shops. The clothes are vedddy, veddy chic. 100% of this store is top designer and brand name items. Chanel Prada, Gucci, Hermes, Valentino, Ferragamo, Tod's and the rest of the gang can be found here. Of course in the most pristine condition, with new things coming in regularly. Get a Prada top for $59 - $250, Chanel from $650-$1800, Ferragamo shoes for $75, Valentino daytime for $150-$350, and a Gucci evening for $250-$1200. They accept consignments until 5pm everyday.

All major credit cards are accepted.

Out of the Closet Thrift
220 E. 81st St. (2nd & 3rd)
212-472-3573

Tues. – Sat. 10-5
Closed August

This store has been around since 1985 and is the first thrift shop created to benefit AIDS charities in NY. 20/20 called them the most crowded store in NY and they are crowded with lots of goodies – great women's and men's clothing, artwork, high-grade bric-a-brac, books. You'll find Armani, Versace, Commes des Garcon, YSL, Elizabeth Arden among their high-end duds and lots of other great brand names too. Tops range anywhere from $3-$200, dresses $20-$600 with great markdowns on items anywhere from 25%-90%. The building itself is also very interesting. It is an 1830's farmhouse with a stable in the back filled with books. They support 50 different AIDS service organizations.

Designer Resale (Consignment)
324 E. 81st St. (1st&2nd)
212-734-3639

M-F 11-7
Thurs. till 8
Sat. 10-6
Sun. 12-5

There are four large rooms to wander through in this store. They carry women's clothing, shoes, handbags, scarves and jewelry. About 50% of this shop is high-end designer clothes with the rest being regular designer and brand names. In addition to the Armani, Chloe, Marc Jacobs, Jill Sander, Fendi, Chanel, Hermes, Moschino which line the racks, they also have a local store (that shall remain nameless) which consigns brand new items sold at consignment store prices. Some of these include Nucci, Industry, Les Chemins, Blumarine, Whistles, C. Puerari, and Theory. Things like Chanel and Prada can go for $300 - $700 with more regular designer clothes at very reasonable prices. Dresses start at $45, slacks $30, suits $95 and blouses $30. They accept consignments everyday until one hour before closing and everything that does not sell is donated to the Salvation Army. The next 2 listings are part of their consignment store "chain", also located on 81st St.

All major credit cards are accepted.

Gentlemen's Designer Resale
322 E. 81st St. (1st & 2nd)
212-734-2739

Children's Resale
303 E. 81st St. (1st & 2nd)
212-734-8897

Both of these shops have the same hours as Designer Resale.

Good-Byes Children's Resale Shop (Consignment)
230 E. 78th St. (2nd & 3rd)
212-794-2301

M-F 11:30-5
Sat. 12-5

This store carries children's clothing, toys, books, and equipment. The clothing ranges from newborn to size 8 and would be considered the better quality high price lines. Many European designers plus the Gap, Ralph Lauren, Jacadi, Petite Bateau can be found here and all are sold for 50% and below the normal retail price. Gap jeans can be gotten for a mere $10 and Petite Bateau rompers for $18. Consignments are accepted by appointment only.

Major credit cards are accepted.

Godmother's League (Thrift)
1459 3rd Ave. (82nd & 83rd)
212-988-2858

M-Sat 10-6
Sun. 12-5
Closed Sun. July & Aug.

This is one of those great, old time thrift shops featuring clothing, home décor and a basement full of furniture. About 25% of the women's clothing is top designers like Armani, Dior, Sonya Rykiel and Matsuda. The rest is high quality merchandise with and without labels we might recognize. Some of the designers carried in the Men's dept are Hugo Boss, Armani and Dior with suits ranging from $60-$125. Women's clothes are very reasonably priced. Dresses range from $20-$35, slacks $10-$25, suits $35-$45 and blouses $10-$20. The charity supported is the West End Day School and they accept donations any day except for Saturday.

Checks are accepted.

Memorial Sloan-Kettering Thrift Shop
1440 3rd Ave. (82nd)
212-535-1250

M-F 10-5:30
Sat. 11-5

This is another great Upper East Side thrift shops with merchandise split 50/50 between clothing and home items, including furniture. Lots of great designer duds here at great prices. Chanel, YSL, Oscar de la Renta and Valentino, to name a few. Many, many new items come in on a regular basis including Berna, Zins, McGlocklin and Brioni. These are direct donations from the manufacturers. Regular slacks range from $10-$35 dresses from $25-$75, suits $35-$75, and blouses $10-$35. Top designer dresses go for $100-$950, suits $125-$850 and blouses $50-$100. There is something for everyone here regardless of your budget or style. Donations are accepted M-F from 9-3:30.

Visa, MC, Amex is accepted.

Spence-Chapin Thrift Shop
1473 3rd Ave. (83rd&84th)
212-737-8448

M-F 10-7
Sat. 10-5
Sun. 12-5

This is another all encompassing thrift shop carrying women's, men's and children's clothing, jewelry, accessories, home décor, furniture, china, glassware, rugs and more. About 50% of the clothing is designer- Armani, Dior, and Jones NY to name a few. Lots of new clothing donated directly from the manufacturers comes in on a regular basis, especially children's. Prices start at $20 for women's and men's clothing and $10 for kids with top designers starting higher. Markdowns are taken on a weekly basis, so be sure to call and find out what's on sale. This store supports the Spence-Chapin service to family and children, which is an adoption agency. Donations are accepted in bags or boxes M-F from 11-4 and Sat. from 11-2. Their sister store is located at 1850 2nd Ave. between 95th & 96th St. This is a larger store with more furniture available.

Visa, MC, Amex, Discover are accepted.
Council Thrift Shop
246 E. 84th St. (2nd & 3rd)
212-439-8373

M-F 11-5:45
Thurs. till 7:45
Sat. 11-4:45
Sun. 12-4:45

This store carries women's clothing and accessories. About 50% of the store is designer clothes with Armani, Valentino and Chanel among many others in attendance. Prices are very reasonable with slacks ranging from $15-$50, dresses $20-$60, suits $40-$100 and blouses $15-$40. This store benefits the National Council of Jewish Women and accepts donations Monday to Friday.

Visa, MC, Amex are accepted

Cancer Care Thrift Shop
1480 3rd Ave. (83rd & 84th)
212-879-9868

M-T-F 11-6
W & Th. 11-7
Sat. 11-4:30
Sun. 12:30-5
Closed Sun. July & August

This store carries women's and men's clothing and some furniture. The clothes are of the highest quality with about 20% of the store being designer names. Some that you may find there are Chanel, Armani, Lacroix, and Louis Feraud. Prices for women's slacks range from $15-$75, dresses $20-$250, suits, $45-$300 and blouses $15-$45. Donations are accepted from Monday to Saturday and this store supports the Cancer Care Social Services Agency, which provides free counseling and some services to cancer patients and their families

MC, Visa, Amex, Checks are accepted.

Bis Designer Resale (Consignment)
1134 Madison Ave. (84th & 85th)
212-396-2760

M-Th. 10-7
F-Sat 10-6

Sun. 12-5

This is an elegant Madison Ave. consignment shop carrying high-end designer clothing and accessories. There is also a small men's department. Gucci, Hermes, Prada, Chanel, Lacroix, St. John can all be found here on a regular basis along with too many others to list. Chanel suits which retail for $2500-$3500 you can grab here for under $600, Hermes which retail for $275 are under $150, and Gucci's which retail for $500 are under $100 here. You can also find many things starting at around $30 and going up, so it's not all 3 digit prices. New items come in constantly and furs are available too. Markdowns are taken on a structured basis with items being reduced 20% after 30 days and 50% after another 30. Consignments are taken anytime.

MC, Visa, Debit Cards are accepted.

Encore (Consignment)
1132 Madison Ave. (84th & 85th)
212-879-2850

This is one of the oldest of the Madison Avenue consignment shops. It's been in business since 1954 and is probably the most well know. There's 2 floors packed with women's, men's and children's designer clothes, shoes, accessories and costume and real fine jewelry. Some of the top designers you will find include Dolce & Gabanna, Hermes, Prada, Armani, Gucci and more. There is a whole Chanel Section and lots of other designer and brand name clothing. You can nab an Armani for $65 up and a Chanel suit for $200 up. Dresses start at $25, with top designers starting at $65. This is a great store with something for everyone. Consignments are accepted Tuesday – Saturday from 10:30 – 5:00.

MC, Visa, Checks are accepted.

Stuyvesant Square Thrift Shop
1704 2nd Ave. (88th & 89th)
212-831-1830

M-Sat. 10-7
Sun. 11-6

This shop carries clothing, housewares, furniture and toys. Three charities are on the same premises including the Goodwill. It is similar to other Goodwill shops.

Spence-Chapin Thrift Shop
1850 2nd Ave. (95th & 96th)
212-426-7643
M & Sat. 10-5
T-F 10-6
Sun. 12-5
See listing for their 3rd Ave. store for information.

West Side
59th – 96th

Off Bdwy Boutique (Consignment)
139 W. 72nd St. (Bdwy & Columbus)
212-724-6713

M-F 10-8
Sat. 11-6
Sun. 1-6

This store is unique in that the front of the store carries new clothing and the back is an upscale consignment shop called Reruns. The owner has informed me that you may find many items that are of the current season in the resale section. It seems that some of her customers buy them up front new and then, after a very brief run on their backs, will bring the garments in for consignment. Sounds good to me! Jill Sanders, Azzedine Alaia, Armani, Prada, Chanel, DKNY and Hermes are some that appear in a starring role here along with a great supporting cast. You can grab Armani slacks from $45-$75, dresses for $40-$200(for an Alaia), and suits for $50 to $150(for a Jill Sanders). Consignments are accepted by appointment only.
All major credit cards are accepted

Housing Works (Thrift)
306 Columbus Ave.
212-579-7566

M-F 11-7
Sat. 10-6
Sun. 12-5

This is a fabulous thrift shop that carries clothing, furniture and home décor. You'll find lots of designer and brand names at great prices.

Major credit cards accepted.

Goodwill Thrift Shop
217 W. 79th St.
212-874-5050

M-Sat. 10-6:45
Sun. 11-6

Clothes, houswares. No furniture.

Salvation Army Thrift Store
268 W. 96th St. (Bdwy & West End)

M-Sat. 10-5:45

Clothing, furniture, electronics, housewares, bric-a-brac.

Above 96th Street

Goodwill Thrift Shop
2196 5th Ave. (135th)
212-862-0020

M-Sat. 10-7
Sun. 11-6
Clothing, furniture and houswares.

Salvation Army Thrift Shop
26 E. 125th St. (Madison)
212-289-9617

M-Sat. 9-5

Clothing, furniture, housewares, books, toys,
electronics.

Brooklyn

Williamsburg
Green Village Used Clothing
460 Driggs Ave. (N.11th)
718-599-4017

M-Thurs. 9-5:30
Fri. 9-2
Sat. Closed
Sun. 10-5:30

The term "thrift warehouse" best describes this 10,000 sq. ft. establishment. Approximately 25% of the store is dedicated to clothing - men's, women's and children's. You'll also find furniture, household items, home décor, fitness equipment, office furniture, bikes and more. Most of the clothing is sold by the pound, at $2 per, with a 10 pound minimum. After 50 lbs. the price goes down to $150 per. There is a better clothing section, which is priced by the piece, with dresses ranging from $10-$25, blouses $3-$9 and coats $12-$60. New York Magazine named this store the "best junk shop in all of NYC". You can get a bedroom set for $200-$400 or a couch for $35-$125. If you're a true bargain hunter, this is the place for you.
Visa, MC is accepted.

Domseys Warehouse Outlet
431 Kent Avenue
718-384-6000

This is another store of gargantuan proportions.
There are 35,000 square feet of used and vintage
clothing to pick through. The staff is very helpful
and have been known to bring customers back
from the brink of shock when they first see how
much there is to choose from. Happy hunting and
pack a lunch!

Bay Ridge

Once Upon a Child
7206 3rd Ave. (72nd & 73rd)
718-491-0300

M-F 10-7
Sat. 11-7
Sun. 12-6

This is a children's resale shop carrying clothing
up to size 10, furniture, equipment and toys.
Clothing ranges from $4-$10. All merchandise is
bought outright and can be brought in for
consideration from 1 hour after opening to 1 hour
before closing.

All major credit cards are accepted.

Salvation Army Thrift Store
3718 Nostrand Ave.
718-648-8930
M-Sat. 10-6

436 Atlantic Ave.
718-8341562
M-Sat. 10-6
Thurs. & Fri. till 7:30

515 5th Ave.
718-832-3960
M-Sat. 10-6

176 Bedford Ave.
718-388-9249
M-Sat. 10-6:15
Thurs. & Fri. till 7:30

239 Flatbush Ave
718-857-7967
M-Sat. 10-6:30
Thurs. & Fri. till 7:30

Clothing, furniture, housewares, bric-a-brac.

981 Manhattan Ave.
718-383-5005
M-Sat. 10-6

Clothing only.

St. Vincent de Paul Thrift Shop
616 Grand Ave. (Leonard & Lorimer)
718-486-8765

M-Sat. 9-3:30

Clothing only.

St Jude Thrift Shop
8706 3rd Ave. (87&88)
718-745-9159

M-Sat. 8-3:45

Clothing and bric-a-brac.

Jamaica

St. Vincent de Paul Thrift
12401 Liberty Ave.
718-835-0361

M-Sat. 9:30-4

Clothing, furniture, housewares.

Burnell's Thrift Shop
17227 Hillside Ave.
718-558-4230

M-F 8-7

This thrift shop carries men's, women's and children's clothing, antiques and electronics.

Astoria

Goodness Gracious Thrift Shop
3013 30th Ave.
718-777-0494

M-F 11-7
Sat. 12-6

You'll find men's, women's and children's clothing and furniture at this store. Donations are accepted at any time.

Cash only.

Flushing

Bayside Thrift Shop
14402 Northern Blvd.
718-460-4141

M-Sat. 11-7
Sun. 12-6

This shop carries men's, women's and children's clothing, housewares, books, and bric-a-brac. A small amount of designer names are available. Dresses go for $6, slacks $4-$5, jackets $6-$7 and blouses $4-$5. The proceeds benefit the Greek Orthodox Church and they accept donations any time.

Discovery Shop
25324 Northern Blvd.
718-631-0296

M-Sat. 10-4

This shop is run by the American Cancer Society and features women's and men's clothing, accessories, housewares, electronics and small appliances. You'll find many designer labels here including Donna Karan, Calvin Klein, Harve Bernard, and Liz Claiborne. Dresses run from $8-$20, slacks $3-$7, jackets $6-$12 and blouses $3-$8. Donations are accepted at any time.

MC, Visa and checks are accepted.

Kathy's Thrift Shop
9812 37th Ave.
718-429-7912

Thurs. – Sat. 9-7
Sun. 10-5

You can find women's, men's and children's clothing here. Dresses range from $5-$8, slacks $1-$4, jackets $3-$4 and blouses $2-$3.

Realty Thrift Shop
10408 Northern Blvd.
718-429-9632

M-Sat. 10-6

You'll find clothing, shoes, household items and bric-a-brac at this shop. Dresses are $4, slacks $3, blouses $2 and jackets $4-$10. This store benefits

the Liberty Baptist Church and they accept
donations at any time.

Programma 2000 (Thrift)
3716 103rd St.
718-476-3086

M-Sun. 11-7

This store carries men's, women's and children's
clothing, furniture and electronics. Clothing sells
for under $10.

Queireo Rodriquez
9118B Corona Ave.
718-760-2805

This shop carries men's, women's and children's
clothing.

Kiddie Re Runs
178-09 Union Tpk. ((178&179)

Tues. – Sat. 9-4:30

You will find new and used children's clothing,
toys and small equipment at this store. They also
have new ladies wool coats and marchasite and
sterling silver jewelry. Used clothing starts at $1,

new dresses go for $8-$9 and jeans $3-$5. All merchandise is bought outright by appointment only and they are very selective.

Sunnyside

Sunnyside Thrift Shop
4625 Greenpoint Ave. (46th & 47th)
718-392-5897

M-Sat. 10-8
Sun. 11-7

This shop carries clothing and household items.

One of a Kind Thrift Shop
4505A Queens Blvd. (45th & 46th)
718-784-0666

M-Sat. 10-8
Sun. 11-7

In this store you will find women's, men's and children's clothing, shoes, books, bric-a-brac, and household items. This are some designer and brand name clothes here such as Liz Claiborne, Valentino, Ann Taylor, Abercrombie & Fitch and the Gap. In men's wear you will find Today's Man, Haggar, Valentino and Cardin. Prices are very reasonable with dresses going for $5-$15, slacks $3-$4, suits $13-$25 and blouses $3-$9.

Men's suits run $15-$30. The proceeds benefit St. Sanorious Cathedral and donations are accepted during store hours.

Bronx

Morris Park Flea Market
1205B Castle Hill Ave.
718-597-5725

Thurs. – Sat. 10-6

You will find contemporary and vintage women's and children's clothing here. You may come across a designer name or two. Dresses start at $5, slacks $5 and suits $25. On Saturday and Sunday they also sell at the Broadway Bazaar on 25th St. in Manhattan.
All major credit cards are accepted.

My Dreams (Thrift)
2769 Webster Ave. (Fordham)
718-561-7122

M-Sat. 9:30-7

This store carries women's, men's and children's clothing, books, antiques and appliances. There are some designer and brand names among the racks such as Calvin Klein and Jordache. Prices range from $2-$10.
Major credit and debit cards are accepted.

Rain Thrift Shop
2211 Powell Ave.
718-597-8560

Tues.- Fri. 9-4

You can find clothing for all members of the family in this store in addition to bric-a-brac and books. Some of the labels you will see are Gap, Michael Jordan, Reebok, and Eddie Bauer. This store benefits the Rain Senior Center and donations are accepted at any time.

Neighborhood House Thrift Shop
466 W. 261st St. (Riverdale Ave.)
718-548-1388

Tues. & Thurs. 10-1
W & F 1-4
Sat. 11-3

This shop carries men's, women's and children's clothing, and bric-a-brac. Every once in a while a designer label will pass through. Dresses, blouses and slacks range from $5-$10 and suits from $10-$12. Children's clothes go up to $5 and men's suits are $10. This store supports the Riverdale Neighborhood House and donations are accepted during store hours.

Salvation Army Thrift Store
1294 Southern Blvd. (Freeman)
718-991-2172
M-Sat. 9-5

2582 3rd Ave. (138th St.)
718-585-5820
M-Sat. 9-5
Clothing, furniture, housewares, bric-a-brac, books electronics.

Mt. Vernon
Pay Last (Thrift)
45 Gramatan Ave. (Sidney & Prospect)
845-667-6007

M-Sat. 10:30-6:30

This store has clothing, shoes, stereos, books, TV's and more.

Yonkers
Salvation Army Thrift Store
29 Pallisade Ave.
914-969-4571

M-Sat. 9:30-5

Clothing, furniture, household items, books electronics and more.

New Rochelle

Humane Society Thrift Shop
313 North Ave. (Garden St, across from Metro North)
914-633-7683

W-Sat. 11-4

This shop has mostly women's clothing, with a small amount of men's and children's available too. You will also find furniture, collectibles, antiques and the like. There is about a 50/50 split between clothing and the other items. They do get many designer and brand name labels such as Versace, Ralph Lauren, Ann Taylor, Gap, Liz Claiborne and Chanel. Dresses sell for $4-$50, pants $2-$7, suits $10 and up and blouses $4-$10. The proceeds go to the Humane Society and donations are accepted at any time. They will also pick up your donations from Westchester, the 5 boros of NYC and western and southern Connecticut.

Federation Thrift Shop
207 North Ave. (Main St.)
914-633-5751

M-F 9:30-5:30
Sat. 10-6

You'll find men's and women's clothing in this store along with furniture, antiques and collectibles. Approximately 50% of the clothing has designer and brand name labels. Some of them include Armani, Gucci, Prada, Jones NY, Dana Buchman, and Donna Karan. They also get new clothing on a regular basis from some of the top NY showrooms. I have seen brand new Bill Blass, Tahari and Ralph Lauren at different times. Dresses range from $10-$2000 for a vintage couture Bob Mackie gown. Slacks go for $5-$75, blouses $5-$100 and suits for $30-$300 for an Armani number. Men's suits can range from $30-$175. This store benefits the United Jewish Appeal of NY and they request you call before you bring in your donations. They will pick up furniture in the tri-state area.

MC, Visa, Discover are accepted.

Larchmont

Golden Shoestring (Thrift & Consignment)
149 Larchmont Ave. (Boston Post Rd.)
914-834-8383

Tues.- Fri. 10-4:30
Sat. 10-5

Women's, men's and children's clothing is the predominant stock of this store, however they do also have jewelry, bric-a-brac and household items

You'll find a good number of designer labels which include Dana Buchman, Jones NY, Talbot's, Ann Taylor and Adrienne Vittadini. Prices are reasonable with dresses going for $6-$20, suits $12-$24, slacks $4-$12 and blouses $4-$8. Men's suits sell for around $25. This store benefits The Junior League of Westchester on the Sound. They are unique in that they accept both donations and consignments, but mostly donations. You can bring in your items at any time as long as they are in good condition.

Checks are accepted.

Scarsdale

Maizie Shop (Consignment)
511 Central Park Ave.
(Directly behind D'errico Jewelers, which is a log cabin)
914-949-1241

Tues. – Sat. 10-5
Thurs. till 7

If longevity counts for anything, the Maize Shop surely wins this one hands down. This shop has been in business since 1942, making it clearly the oldest consignment store in Westchester County, if not all of New York. They carry women's clothing, accessories, handbags, shoes and jewelry. Their stock is almost all top designer and brand name labels. You'll find St. John, Escada, Armani, Ann Klein, Eileen Fisher, Ann Taylor, BCBG, and Ellen Tracy on a regular basis. Dresses range from $19-$129 with top designers going for up to $299. Suits go for $39-$149 with a Chanel or St. John from $299-$399. You can get a blouse for $10-$39 and slacks for $16-$39 with the top labels going up to $79. They cater to all women with sizes ranging from 2-22. Consignments are accepted by appointment only and must be newly cleaned and pressed.

Visa, MC and Checks are accepted.

Dobbs Ferry

Affordables (Children's Consignment)
10 Main St. (Walnut)
914-693-3610

M-Sat. 10-5
Thurs. till 6

This shop carries children's clothing, equipment, toys, books, games and maternity clothes. Mom's can shop in peace as this is a child-friendly environment. There are toys and games to keep the kids amused while mommy shops. You'll find Gap, Children's Place and Gymboree items among their racks at very good prices. Gap pants range from $6.50-$7.50, shirts $5.50-$6.50 and sweaters

$12. Consignments are taken by appointment only.

All major credit cards, checks are accepted.

Now & Again (Consignment)
123A Main St. (Oak St.)
914-693-7841

M-F 10-4
Sat. 10-5

This store specializes in women's clothing shoes and accessories. You'll find lots of designer and brand name labels here including Armani, Escada, Calvin Klein, Jones NY, Talbot's, Ann Klein, and Bloomingdales. Average prices are $12-$35 for dresses, $18-$25 for suits, $8-$15 for blouses and $12-$18 for pants. Top designer names can go for more. They also have a good selection of the larger sizes included in their stock and all of their shoes are brand new. The proceeds from this store benefits the Community Hospital at Dobb's Ferry and the Clearview School. They accept consignments by appointment only.

Checks are accepted.

White Plains

St. Bartholomew's Thrift Shop
60 Sterling Ave. (Prospect St.)
914-949-5611
This is a shop that carries high end women's clothing, shoes, accessories, bric-a-brac and a small amount of men's and children's clothing. Lots of designer and brand name labels are to be had here at very, very low prices. You will be find everything from Armani, Prada, and de la Renta to Liz Claiborne, Banana Republic and Gap. Dresses go for $7-$10, slacks $3-$4, suits $10 and blouses $3. They also get brand new merchandise from top stores, which shall remain nameless (hint-you'll find them at The Westchester). This store benefits outreach programs in White Plains. They accept donations anytime, but please call first.

Port Chester

Salvation Army Thrift Shop
36 N. Main St. (Westchester Ave.)
914-939-1620

M-Sat. 9:30-5:30
Thurs. & Fri. till 7:30

Clothing, furniture, electronics, books and more.

Piermont

Tappan Zee Thrift Shop
454 Piermont Ave. (Ferdon)
845-359-5753

Tues, Thurs, Fri & Sat. 10-4

You'll find women's, men's, and children's clothing, household items, books and bric-a-brac at this shop. There are a lot of brand names here and some designer wear. Some that you will see are DKNY, Gap, and Old Navy. Most items are priced from $3-$10. The proceeds benefit 10 different area charities and they accept donations from 10:30-3:00.

Checks are accepted.

Nyack

Nyack Hospital Thrift Shop
117 Main St. (Franklin)
845-358-7933

Tues.- Sat. 10-3:45

This store carries women, men's and children's clothing. Prices range from $3-$14 with an occasional designer label popping up. This shop benefits Nyack hospital and they ask that you bring in donations before 3:00.

Chappaqua

Discovery Shop (Thrift)
400 King St. (Rt. #117)
914-238-4900

M-F 10-4:30
Sat. 10-1

This is another of those fabulous American Cancer Society thrift shops with a large amount of designer and brand name clothes at great prices. Armani, Escada, Donna Karan, Calvin Klein, Liz Claiborne, Jones NY, Villager and more pass through here on a regular basis. Dresses run from $10-$50, suits $15-$50, slacks $8-$25, and blouses $8-$20. Men's suits go for $30-$50. You can bring in your donations until 3:00.

Visa, MC, Amex is accepted.

Opportunity Shop (Thrift & Consignment)
61 N. Greeley Ave. (King)
914-238-4420

M-F 10-4

This is both a consignment and thrift shop, which carries women's and men's clothing, accessories,

jewelry and bric-a-brac. You'll find some designer
and brand name duds such as Ralph Lauren,
Donna Karan, Armani, Gap, Banana Republic and
LL Bean. Dresses range from $10-$35, suits $15-
$45, and slacks $6-$20. Men's suits go for $25-
$35. The proceeds benefit the Sisterhood of
Temple Beth-El's local charities. Donations are
accepted anytime and consignments are taken from
10:00-12:00.

Checks are accepted.

Bedford

Rummage Round Shop(Thrift)
16 Banksville Ave. (North St.)
914-234-6987

W-Sat. 10-4

This shop carries clothing, kitchenware, books,
toys, bric-a-brac and small furniture. You'll find a
few designer labels among the clothes such as
Tommy Hilfiger and Ralph Lauren. Prices range
from $2-$35. Donations are accepted at any time.
Checks are accepted.

Greenwich

Merry Go Round (Thrift)
38 Arch St. (Greenwich Ave.)
203-869-3155

T-Sat. 10-3

This shop carries a wide variety of merchandise ranging from clothing for the family to furniture and everything in between. You will find a large amount of designer and brand name clothes including Chanel, Gucci, Ferragamo, Pucci, Valentino and Scassi. Dresses go for $15-$50, slacks $8-$15, suits $25-$45 and blouses $5-$12. They also get new items regularly. The proceeds benefit the Muse Senior Residence and they will accept donations any day from 10-2.

Checks are accepted.

ELDE Thrift Shop
522 E. Putnam Ave. (Indian Field Rd)
203-869-0464

M-Sat. 9-4:30
You'll find men's and women's clothing and housewares in this shop. About on quarter of the

clothing is designer or brand name. St. John and
Armani stop in every now and then. Dresses range
from $10-$125, suits $25-$150, slacks and blouses
$8-$25. This store benefits The Education
Learning Development Center and they accept
donations every day from 10-3.

Checks are accepted.

Rummage Room (Thrift)
191 Sound Beach Ave. (Post Rd, US #1)
203-637-1875

M-F 10-5
Sat. 10-1

This store carries men, women's and children's
clothing and household items. You will find
designer wear here, such as Ann Klein, DKNY,
Dana Buchman, Ann Taylor and Ferragamo.
Prices range from $6-$20 for most items. The
proceeds support a number of local charities and
donations are accepted M-Th. 9-5, Fri. 9-1 and Sat.
9:30-1.

Checks are accepted.

Stamford

Laurel House Thrift Shop
501 Summer St. (Spring)
203-323-0808

M-F 9-4
Sat. 9-3

This store has clothing for the family, furniture and household goods. You may come across a designer name now and again. This store supports charities for the mentally ill and addicted and accepts donations at any time.
Checks are accepted.

Darien

Double Exposure Consignment
1091 Post Rd. (Exit 11 off I-95)
203-655-5799

M-Sat. 10-5
Th. till 7
Sun. 12-4

You will find mostly women's clothing at this store, however there is also some furniture, collectibles and artwork to rummage through. The clothing is anything from Banana Republic to Chanel. Dresses range anywhere from $30-$300, suits $48-$128, blouses $24-$40 and slacks $20-$60. They have a structured system for a markdown with prices reduced 20% after 30 days and 50% after 60 days. Anything left over after that is donated to "Dress for Success".

Visa, MC, Amex and checks (with CT ID) are accepted.

Darien Community Thrift Shop
996 Post Rd. (Corbin Dr.)
203-655-4552

T-F 10-4:30
Sat. 10-4

This store has a 50/50 split between clothing and household items. There is a boutique section where the designer and brand names are stashed. You can see Armani, Donna Karan, Ann Klein and Fendi to name a few. Prices range anywhere from $6-$150. The proceeds go to the Darien Community Association and donations are accepted Tues, Thurs. and Sat. 10-2.

Visa and MC are accepted.

_____Chapter 7_____

Sale Events

Most, if not all sale events featuring pre-owned clothing are held to benefit a particular charity. So that means with every penny you spend you are doing a good deed (accruing merit for the Buddhists among us). Yippee! Shopping without guilt! Individuals or designers, stores and manufacturers donate all of the merchandise sold. These events are loads of fun and competition can get wild. Get there early, as there is usually a line. Don't be intimidated by those aggressive shoppers. If you find yourself getting physical with someone over a Fendi bag marked $20, just think of it as "boxing for broads" and go for it! (*JUST* a joke)

Long Island

Locust Valley

Grenville-Baker Boys and Girls Club Annual Clothing Sale
135 Forest Ave.
516-759-5437

Every April, for the past 37 years, the gymnasium of this club is filled to the rafters with gently used upscale clothing, shoes, accessories, jewelry, furs, bric-a-brac and household items. This is an incredible sale that goes on for a week and a half, and it could take you that long to pore through all that is available here. Some of the designer labels I have seen here are Chanel, Dior, Claude Montana, Oscar de la Renta, Ferragamo, St. John, Armani, Scassi, Ungaro and on and on. There are far too many to list. I picked up the most beautiful $300 Trussardi leather bag for $70. It was in perfect condition and I was ecstatic. Furs go for $300-$600. They've had Chanel suits that sold for $100-$150, Prada purses for $20 and men's brand new designer ties for $1-$5. Local stores also donate new items to this sale. Prices start at $.50 and go to up. There is something in every price range and style. This is a bargain hunter's paradise. And if that weren't enough, they have a special "Donor's Day". When you donate items to this sale you get a ticket to shop on the day before the sale opens to the public. Yippeee!! It's lots of fun and lots of great deals. Plus the proceeds also benefit a very good cause. Call to get on their mailing list.

Visa, MC, Amex and checks with ID are accepted.

Manhattan

The Posh Sale
New York Lighthouse for the Blind
111 E.59th St. (Mad. & Park)
212-821-9200

This once a year event happens in May and is absolutely phenomenal. This not to be missed extravaganza features new and gently used clothing (and we do mean gently, nothing worn looking is accepted), jewelry, accessories, furs and home décor donated by NY's crème de la crème. Prices start at $5 with top designer clothes start at $15. Many designers donate new items. This year Liz Claiborne, Geoffrey Beene (over 300 pieces), Kenneth Cole, Kasper, Starington (Silk blouses and dresses) have all donated new items. Liz priced $15 -$40, Beene $125 - $275(gowns). The "pre-owned" category includes Armani, Escada, Donna Karan, Givenchy, Yves St. Laurent, Ralph Lauren and too many more to list. Get an Armani suit for as low as $125, Ferragamo shoes for $40, furs $300 and up. There is a celebrity rack, with items donated by the famous and infamous and now, for a second year, a Vintage section. I assure you everything is at a mere fraction of what you would pay in the stores. I still get compliments on things I bought at these sales 15 years ago!

You can call them or go to their website for information on this. The address is http://www.lighthouse.org/calendar_main.htm

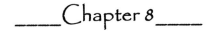

_____Chapter 8_____

Chain Thrift Stores

Something new has appeared on the scene over the last couple of years, namely thrift stores as large as a supermarket. There are five that I have found scattered over Long Island. They have the feel of a K-Mart with all used merchandise. The prices for clothing are very low with most items selling for $1-$12. There are lots and lots to rummage through and every once in a while you might come across a designer or brand name.

Savers
W. Hempstead
188 Hempstead Tpk.
516-489-1661

E. Meadow
2575 Hempstead Tpk.
516-579-1466

M-Sat. 9-9
Sun. 10-6

Visa, MC, Discover, Debit, and checks are accepted.

Northern Thrift
Huntington Station
2035 New York Ave. (Rt. #110)
631-673-4790

M 9:30-6
T-Sat. 9:30-9
Sun. 11-7

MC, Visa, and checks are accepted

Island Thrift
Brentwood
700 Suffolk Ave
631-231-0460

M-Sat 9:30-8
Sun. 10-7
MC, Visa are accepted

Selden
Selden Thrift
614 Middle Country Rd. (Bluepoint Ave)
631-736-3979

M 9:30-6
T-Sat. 9:30-9
Sun. 11-7

MC, Visa, and checks are accepted

Northshore Thrift
Port Jefferson Station
544 Jefferson Plaza on Rt. # 112
631-642-0022

M 9:30-6
T-Sat. 9:30-9
Sun. 11-7

MC, Visa, and checks are accepted

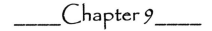

_____Chapter 9_____

Vintage Shops

Vintage stores carry clothing, accessories, shoes and jewelry from the Victorian era to the early 1980's. Yikes! If my old clothes are considered vintage, what does that make me? Well...Praise the Lord, and pass the Botox.

Some stores will have stock from all eras, while others will specialize in a certain period. The prices for these garments vary as much as contemporary clothing. I myself am partial to vintage items from the 30's and 40's, and as time passes these pieces become harder to find and more expensive to purchase. They are available though. What is very popular right now are couture from the 60's and 70's. Halston, Courreges, Pauline Trigere, are all very hot. So if you have one hanging in your closet and are not emotionally attached to it, you can probably take it to an upscale consignment or vintage shop, where it will be welcomed.

Long Island

Port Jefferson

Vintage & Vogue
134 Main St.
631-331-1864

This store has new clothing and vintage from the 50's and 60's.

Manhattan

Below Houston

What Comes Around Goes Around
351 W. Bdwy (Broome & Grand)
212-343-9303

M-Sun. 11-7
You can find vintage and dead stock designer, military, western, denim and leather clothing and accessories here for both women and men. They also carry their own line, WGACA, which is reconstructed vintage t-shirts, motorcycle jean jackets and grommeted jeans that range from $35-$300. They are known for the largest collection of

vintage denim in the city. There are literally thousands of pieces of Levi's, Wrangler's and Lee's to choose from. Jeans can start at $45 and go up to $1000 for a pair of Levi's Biggie XX. Some of the designers you can find are Courreges, Pucci, YSL, and Alaia. Designer dresses start at $100 and you can get a 2-piece Courreges with jacket for $1000. They also have a 6000 sq. ft. warehouse at 13-17 Laight St. (St. John's Lane & Varrick St.) which has over 50,000 items. Whereas the store carries the clothing of the season, the warehouse encompasses all seasons. In addition to selling to retail customers they cater to every asset of the design industry. Costumers, designers and stylists all come here to glean inspiration, rent pieces or even get a loan. The warehouse is available by appointment only. All of their merchandise is bought outright.

All major credit cards are accepted.

Resurrection Vintage
217 Mott St. (Spring & Prince)
212-625-1374

M-Sat. 11-7
Sun. 12-7

What you will find at this store is high-end designer clothes for the 1960's - 1970's. Halston,

Courreges, Pucci, Gucci, Thea Porter, Ozzie Clark and YSL are all frequent visitors. Dresses range from $100-$1000, suits the same, jeans start at $100 and a pair of YSL black slacks can go for $400-$500. They buy their merchandise outright and you must make an appointment to bring in your clothing.

All major credit cards are accepted.

Foley & Corinna
108 Stanton St.
212-529-2338

M-F 1-8
S&S 12-8

Although this store carries items from the Victorian era up to the 70's, most of their stock is from the 60's and 70's. They specialize in everyday wearable vintage. Prices range from $35-$200.

Major credit cards are accepted.

David Owens Vintage Clothing
154 Orchard St. (Rivington & Stanton)
212-677-3301

You will find men and women's clothing from the 40's to the 80's along with accessories and fine leathers and suedes. They specialize in unique vintage furs in mint condition, rayon and cotton Hawaiian shirts $25-$295 and a large selection of 1940's neckties, including peek-a-boos. You can also find their wares everyday at the Flea Market at Broadway and E. 4th Street and on Saturday's and Sunday's at The Annex on Sixth Avenue between 25th and 26th Streets.

Visa and MC are accepted.

Vintage Eyewear of NYC
917-721-6546
http://www.vintage-eyewear.com

I found this dealer at the Manhattan Vintage Clothing Show and was so impressed with their unique stock that, although they sell only at shows and from their website, I decided to include them in this book. They specialize in eyewear from as far back as the 1700's up to the 1970's. They have a vast collection of new old stock from the 30's to 70's, which includes many couture collectibles. You can pick out a frame and have them do the lens work from your custom prescription or sunglasses. I absolutely loved what they have to offer and have never seen anyone quite like them before. I'm not alone in my awe, as they have a client list of top designers, fashion houses and museums curators worldwide.

East Side
Houston - 14th

Andy's CheePees
691 Bdwy (3rd & 4th)
212-420-5980

M-Sat. 11-9
Sun. 12-8

This store carries vintage clothing from the 1920's -1980's. Some of the things you'll find are prom dresses, tuxedos, t-shirts, leather goods jeans. This store targets the younger crowd, from the teens to late 20's. Prom dresses can be had for $65-$125, plaid pants go for $30-$55, jeans $30-$85, and t-shirts $8-$55. Women's leather items go for $45-$135 and men's $75-$350. They buy their merchandise outright.

All major credit cards are accepted.

Eye Candy
329 Lafayette St. (Bleeker & Houston)
212-343-4275

M-Sun. 12-8

This unique shop specializes in vintage accessories - handbags, shoes, scarves, hats, jewelry and watches. They also carry some selective pieces of clothing. A lot of the jewelry is collectable designer pieces, however there *is* something for everyone. Some of the names you can find in jewelry are Hattie Carnegie, Miriam Haskell, Givenchy, Trifari, Schiaparelli, and Pucci. In the shoe department you will find La Rose and Charles Jourdan. Chanel, Pucci and Dior scarves can be had as well as Pucci and Gucci dresses. Lots of beaded and mesh purses from the 1920's abound along with Gucci, Chanel and Vuitton from the 70's. Prices start at $25 and go up to $350 for jewelry, $150 for shoes and $300 for handbags. All merchandise is bought outright.

All major credit cards and checks are accepted.

Screaming Mimi's
382 Lafayette St. (4th St.)
212-677-6464

M-Sat. 12-8
Sun. 12-6

This downtown landmark has been around since 1978. They carry women's and men's clothing ranging from the 1940's to 1980's, however everything is in such good condition, at first glance you might not realize it's vintage. The prices downstairs are very affordable ranging from $16-

$60 and a balcony of designer clothes is in the works. Dresses start at $20 and for a 40's evening dress or 60's beaded number you'll pay up to $125. There is a small selection of suits ranging form $55-$110. You can get a blouse for $20 and they go up to $78 for a 60's beaded or embroidered peasant blouse. Everything is bought outright.

All credit card are accepted.

Angela's Vintage Boutique
330 E.11th St. (1st & 2nd)
212-475-1571
212-475-3150

T-F 12-8
S&S 1-8

This store stocks clothing and accessories from the Victorian era to the 50's. They specialize in gowns from the 20's and 30's, with lots of fancy lace and chiffon everywhere you look. There are items to fit all budgets with prices starting at $50 and going up to $2000 for a handmade Brandenburg or $1500 for a Worth jacket.

All major credit cards accepted.

Cheap Jack's Vintage Clothing
841 Bdwy (13th & 14th)
212-995-0403

M-Sat. 11-8
Sun. 12-7

You will find 3 floors of men, women's and teen's clothing ranging from the 1970's and before. They don't focus on labels here; the condition of the garment is what's important. You'll come across Hawaiian and bowling shirt's that range from $35-$85 with a rare 1920's Hawaiian shirt going for as much as $500. There's a selection of vintage dresses from the 20's-40's ranging from $1 all the way to $300 for a spectacular 40's number. Another one of their specialties is vintage t-shirts, especially of the "rock" variety going for $.50 to $85 for a 1970's Led Zeppelin artifact. Antique beaded purses go for $125 and jeans average $15-$140 with a first edition pair of Levi's for $5000. Men's suits start at $125 and go up. There are even price tags that read $0 if purchased with another item. They buy all of their merchandise outright.

All major credit cards and travelers checks are accepted.

West Side
Houston - 14th

Cherry
19 8th Ave. (12th)
212-924-7131

M-Sun. 12-8

This vintage store features designer and couture clothing from the 1950's – 1980's. Their style is quite funky with lots of unique leather pieces abounding. There is a large selection of designer shoes, and they also carry coats and accessories. Some of the designers you can find there are Pucci, Alaia and Courreges. Grab a Pucci dress for $650, a Diane Von Furstenberg for $125 or a suit for $100-$800. They buy their clothing outright.

West Side
14th - 59th

The Family Jewels
130 W. 23rd St. (6th & 7th)
212-633-6020

Sun -Wed. 11-7
Thurs. - Sat. 11-8

Vogue, Elle and In Style magazines have all named this store as one of the best vintage shops in the country. They've been in business for 20 years and there are 2000 sq. feet of men's and women's clothing and accessories from the Victorian era to the 1970's, with the predominant years being the 50's and 60's. You'll find everything from 1920's flapper dresses, to 40's rayon numbers to the top designers of the 70's. Hattie Carnegie, Chanel, Pauline Trigere, and Pucci are some of the labels you will see. The price range is as wide as the selection going anywhere from $10 - $600, so there is truly something for everyone. Cocktail dresses start at $75, 40's dresses $15 and up, women's suits $150 and up and men's suits $250 and up. Their costume jewelry, handbag, shoe and lingerie collections are also quite extensive. Find those great Lucite or beaded purses here. Many major designers and Broadway theaters use this store as a resource. They buy outright at wholesale prices and you must make an appointment for this. They have a website too! Check it out at http://www.familyjewelsnyc.com.

All major credit cards and checks are accepted

Deco Etc.
@ The Showplace
40 W. 25th St. (5th & 6th)
Lower Level, Gallery 119

212-620-0827

S&S 8:30 – 5:30
Weekdays by appointment
212-683-6335

This store specializes in Art Deco items from the 30's to the 50's. They have a large selection of extremely unique handbags and jewelry from this era. You can find those fabulous Lucite handbags and accessories along with beaded purses and Bakelite jewelry. There are figural wicker bags in the shape a monkey, fish or dog and those way cool scenic straw bags. Prices can range anywhere from $50 to $10,000 for an especially unique and rare item. Handbags usually go for $85-$300 and Bakelite jewelry from $65 up. They also carry lighting and decorative objects from the era. All major credit cards and checks are accepted.

Quincy Kirsch
@ International Antique Center
30 W. 28th St. (5th & 6th)
917-414-4598

Th – F 1-5
Sat. Sun. Dawn – 5 at Garage Flea Market, 106 W. 25th St.

You'll find items from the 1800's to the 1960's in this establishment, with most coming from the

20's-50's. The clothing here is the fun and kitchy type, things like circle skirts and the like, more everyday vintage than fancy schmancy. Prices range from $20 up to $500.

All major credit cards and checks are accepted.

Lucille's Antique Corner
127 W. 26th St. (6th & 7th)
212-691-1041

Wed. 12-7
Sat. - Sun. 9-7:30

Over 60% of this 3500 sq. foot store are dedicated to clothing. You will find vintage and designer vintage women's and men's items. The rest of the space is antiques and linens. Chanel, Oscar de la Renta, Rossi, Bill Blass and Ann Klein are some of the designer names that pass through. There is an extensive selection of shoes that are almost all designer brands. Dresses start at $25 and can go up to $600 for a top designer. Suits range from $100-$250. They buy all merchandise outright.

All major credit cards and checks are accepted

West Side
59th - 96th

Allan & Suzi (Vintage)
416 Amsterdam Ave. (80th St.)
212-724-7445

M-Sun. 12-7

Eveningwear tops the bill in this shop, which has been in business since 1987. They carry vintage from the 1950's-1970's and current items from the past 3 years. Lots and lots of designer labels are found here both in vintage and contemporary. Some of the names you'll see are YSL, Courreges(60's), Lacroix, Valentino, Dior, Paco Rabanne, Chanel, Ungaro, and Gaultier, They also have accessories and beautiful collection of vintage jewelry. There is something in every price range with items starting at $10. They accept consignments at any time. They also have a store in Asbury Park, NJ at 711 Cookman Ave.

All major credit cards are accepted.

Brooklyn

Park Slope

Almost New Clothing
68 St. Mark's Ave. (6th & Flatbush)
718-398-8048

M-Sun. 12-7
Closed Wed.

You'll find vintage women's and men's clothing, jewelry, accessories and shoes, and contemporary haute couture items in this shop. The stock can range from the 1930's -1970's with even a few pieces from the 20's and before. About 30% of the clothing have designer labels such as Versace, Armani, Moshcino, and Chanel. This store is a favorite haunt for stylists and designers as well as the personal shoppers of many top celebs. Prices are affordable with dresses averaging from $15-$35 and going up to $100-$150 for top designers. Suits go for $35-$45, 40's bags $18-$95, and hats $10-$35. You can sell your items outright to this store,
however furs will be taken on consignment.
Please call for an appointment to do either.

All major credit cards and checks are accepted.

Hootie Couture
179 Berkley Pl. (7th & 8th)
718-857-1977

M-Sun. 11-7:30

This shop carries vintage clothing, handbags, shoes, costume jewelry and accessories from the 1940's to 1980's. You'll even find some houseware items here. The name of the store is a bit of a play on words, reflecting the everyday style
of clothes found here combined with the owner's name, Allison Houtte. You will see designer labels mixed into the racks, such as Bonnie Cashin, Enid Collins, Chanel, Ralph Lauren. Dresses can range anywhere from $18-$65, slacks $1-$150, blouses $15-$35, jewelry $5-$45 and handbags from $18-$80. All the merchandise in this store is bought outright in bulk from estate sales and the like.

Visa, MC, Discover, Debit Cards are accepted

Westchester

White Plains
Vintage by Stacey Lee
305 Central Ave., Suite 4
914-328-0788

Open by appointment only.

This store carries items from the 1900's to the 1970's. They specialize in designer clothing and accessories such as Hermes, Gucci, Pucci and Dior. Their collection of handbags from these eras is quite extensive. Every price range can be found

Checks are accepted.

Southwestern Connecticut

Greenwich

Sophia's Great Dames Vintage
1 Liberty Way (Elm & Lewis)
203-869-5990

M-Sat. 10-5:30

This is an antique shop that has a second floor full of vintage clothing. The year's range from the Victorian Era to the 1960's and you will find many vintage couture numbers. Gucci, Balenciaga, Molyneax, Jacques Fath, Worth and Dior are some of the labels you will see. Dresses average $25-$100, but if you're looking for rare Chanel from the 40's be prepared to shell out a few thousand. Suits start at $25 and go up to $400 for a 60's Courreges or Halston. Blouses can range from $10-$100. They both accept consignments and buy outright, but call before you bring your things in.

Major credit cards and checks are accepted.

_____Chapter 10_____

Vintage Sale Events

Throughout the year different companies host Vintage Clothing Shows. At these events, anywhere from 40 to 125 dealers will gather to sell their wares. You will find all the different types of specialties you would have to travel far and wide to see, all under one roof.

Manhattan Vintage Clothing Show
@ Metropolitan Pavilion
110 W. 19th St. (6th & 7th)
New York, NY
518-434-4312

This show is held four times per year, April, June, September and November at NYC's Metropolitan Pavilion. Forty to fifty vendors from 14 states come here to exhibit, so whether you are looking for couture gowns from the 40's, poodle skirts from the 50's or funky duds from the 60's you are bound to find it along with lots more. Every era is represented from the 1800's to the 1980's as well as every style and budget. You will find men's and women's clothing, shoes, accessories, jewelry and eyewear. This show is a true delight to visit for shoppers and spectators alike. Anyone interested in fashion history will marvel walking through the aisles, but I dare you to make it out the door without making a purchase. *That's* nearly impossible! Admission is $20. Find the dates on the website http://www.manhattanvintage.com.

Westchester County Center Vintage Clothing, Jewelry & Textiles Show & Sale
@ The Westchester County Center
Tarrytown Rd. & Rte. 100
White Plains, NY
914-248-4646

These shows are held three times per year at the Westchester County Center. Up to 120 vendors exhibit here and as the name suggests you will find everything from clothing to textiles to estate and costume jewelry. Every era, style and budget can be found here and they also have prizes for the patron who comes dressed in the most authentic vintage outfit. You can win $250, $100 or $50. Oooooo! Imagine having that extra cash to spend. A shopaholics dream day! Admission is $7 and you can get the dates from their website http://www.mavencompany.com .

Antique Textile Vintage Fashions Show & Sale
@Host Hotel
Rte. 20
Sturbridge, MA
207-439-2334

Although this show is beyond the New York area I have decided to include it since it kicks off Brimfield Week, a legend among vintage shoppers everywhere. It is held three times per year on the Monday before the start of the Brimfield shows. Brimfield, a small New England town, hosts what Arts & Antique Weekly called "the mother of all outdoor fairs". Rather then one complete show, this event is more than 20 shows which open in a sequential fashion beginning at daybreak on Tuesday and running through the week. The clothing and textile show is held indoors at the Host Hotel and runs for one day only. Anywhere from 90 – 150 exhibitors from 20 states and 6 countries will show here. Country Homes Antique Magazine has written - "This show kicks off Brimfield week and for some our staff, it's the best part of the week." Expect to find tapestries, costumes, coverlets, homespun, samplers, sewing items, hooked rugs, needlepoint, old wallpaper, antique fans, leather suitcases, curtain hardware, old buttons, beaded purses, antique jewelry, brocades, vintage clothing from all periods, doll clothes, hats, shoes, buttons, quilts, fabric, laces, trims and linens.

Notes